The Social Meaning
of Midwifery

Related titles from Macmillan

The Midwifery Practice Series
eds Jo Alexander, Valerie Levy and Sarah Roch

Antenatal care
Intrapartum care
Postnatal care

Theory for Midwifery Practice, Rosamund Bryar

The Social Meaning of Midwifery

Sheila C. Hunt
Head of Midwifery Education
Department of Nursing and Midwifery
University of Wales, Swansea

and

Anthea Symonds
Lecturer in Social Policy
University of Wales, Swansea

WQ 150

MACMILLAN

First published 1995 by
MACMILLAN PRESS LTD
Houndmills, Basingstoke, Hampshire RG21 2XS
and London
Companies and representatives
throughout the world

ISBN 0–333–60877–1

A catalogue record for this book is available
from the British Library.

10   9   8   7   6   5   4   3
04   03   02   01   00

Copy-edited and typeset by Povey–Edmondson
Okehampton and Rochdale, England

Printed in Great Britain by
Antony Rowe Ltd
Chippenham, Wiltshire, England

Dedicated to the memory of my much-loved sister, Maureen Elizabeth, who died on 31 December 1993, aged 32 years, mother of Sean, Fay and Madeleine.

SHEILA C. HUNT

Contents

List of Figures and Tables

☐ **Figures**

☐ **Tables**

Foreword

How do we interpret our world? How do we make sense of what is going on around us in an unfamiliar environment as a new member of staff, a student or as a woman making use of maternity services? How do we come to an understanding of the performance that as midwives, students, childbearing women or medical staff in which we are being asked to participate, where the scenes, roles, plot, characters and script have been largely 'prepared earlier'? Sheila Hunt and Anthea Symonds in this book have given us the tools to be able to undertake this interpretation and have provided a means of analysing the complex world of maternity care. The authors have undertaken an extremely valuable task in that they have, in the partnership of their writing, linked for us theory and practice. The descriptions by Sheila Hunt of the maternity units she studied will ring true for many readers. Yes, there will be nuances of differences for different midwives – from my experience I miss reference to knitting and to the particular type of humour found in maternity units!

But Sheila Hunt and Anthea Symonds have done a more important job than describing and analysing the work in these units – they have opened our eyes. How often have we stood back and observed the activities, notices, behaviours, talk, use of space and other factors in the world of the maternity unit? How often have we considered the extent to which our basic concepts about midwifery care are demonstrated in the social world of which we are a part, which we have helped to create and thus have the potential to change? The authors make clear, though, that such description has to be placed in the wider framework of society and the many factors which have influenced the role of the midwife and the provision of maternity services. They provide a comprehensive and challenging picture of that context which will be as disturbing to some readers as the description of the labour ward activities will be to others.

This, then, is not a book to be approached lightly – possibly it needs some sort of health warning. As with another, very different book, readers should be warned 'this book will change your life'! The authors provide evidence and analysis which challenge many of the complacent images that midwives hold of themselves and the care that they provide. By doing this they make a very important contribution to midwifery. At a time when midwives are being asked to examine their fundamental beliefs as changes are introduced to ensure greater continuity, choice and control, this book provides a means of understanding the present world of midwifery practice. It is only when everyone, including midwives, childbearing women, doctors, sociologists and managers, have an understanding of the past and present factors affecting maternity services that effective and realistic change can be made to these services. I urge everyone involved in the provision of maternity care, in receipt of maternity care and in research and teaching related to maternity care to read this book. Maternity services may never be the same again!

Swansea   ROSAMUND BRYAR

Preface

This book is based on an ethnographic study of two hospital labour wards. The research was undertaken by Sheila Hunt in the late 1980s and early 1990s. She was a clinical midwife and more latterly a teacher of midwifery. Anthea Symonds became interested in both the study and in midwives when she was involved in joint planning of the first pre-registration midwifery education programme in Wales. Anthea is a sociologist with particular interest in occupational cultures and health policies. She read the first ethnographic study and was excited by its sociological potential and felt that there would be wider interest in the content.

At a series of successful 'double acts' at conferences and study days the ideas and concepts of the book were developed and refined. There was a strong feeling that this book would not go away despite the efforts they made to ignore it and their often waning interest in the topic. In 1993 they were forced to put pen to paper. Anthea wrote Chapters 1 and 2, while the remaining chapters were written by Sheila and are based on her research. The content will be controversial and may even upset some midwives. It appears that it is a tale that has to be told. Such studies can make uncomfortable reading but there is no doubt that exploring aspects of care in this detail cannot but help thinking midwives to consider midwifery practice more deeply and improve upon the care of women in childbirth.

SHEILA C. HUNT
ANTHEA SYMONDS

Acknowledgements

We would like to thank:

- The women in the study who were willing to share their experience of birth.
- The midwives of Valley Maternity Hospital who were so willing to cooperate and eager to talk about themselves and their work.
- The midwives and students who at study days and conferences urged us to write this book because they believed that by looking at ourselves we could learn so much and improve care for women.
- The midwifery lecturers and Director of the Department of Nursing and Midwifery for their support.
- Paul Atkinson and Anne Murcott of the University College, Cardiff, who taught Sheila to be an ethnographer.
- Ruth Davies (WNB), who taught Sheila never silently to tolerate poor standards.
- And finally our long suffering families, David, Ruth and Thomas Hunt and Dr Keith Lewis.

SHEILA C. HUNT
ANTHEA SYMONDS

Introduction

This book is about midwives, midwifery and women. It explores the social meaning of midwifery, considers birth as it happened in many British maternity hospitals in the late 1980s and offers an opportunity for past, present and future midwives to analyse aspects of their practice. Above all this is a study of women at work, and as such should prove of interest to sociologists and feminists.

The ethnographic study of two particular groups of midwives at work in two hospitals in the very recent past (1989) attempts to unravel their constructed occupational identity. It must be stressed that we are not setting up a generalist model of midwifery or claiming a universal theoretical understanding of what it means to be a midwife which would be applicable to everyone working anywhere. This is in the nature of an exploration into an understanding of the ways in which an identity of an occupational group is constructed in everyday practice. The study looks at the ways in which real women act in real situations in the everyday 'normal' hospital practice of midwifery. Evidently, this is not an account of a universal experience and some midwives will read this and fail to recognise any familiarity within the text, but equally there are many others to whom the situations, language and circumstances described here will strike a chord.

This book is in two main parts, the first part will be a 'scene-setting' exercise wherein the historical, political and social background to the construction of this specific occupational group and the site of its working practice is set out as well as a description of the methodology involved. The second part consists of the ethnographic study of the labour wards, which must be read within the theoretical framework set out in the first two chapters.

■ Searching for social meaning

The fundamental argument underlying this book is that descriptions of an occupation such as 'midwife' have no intrinsic meaning of their own. To be a midwife is a cultural and historical experience. This experience will differ from culture to culture and over time. To be a midwife in a Bronze Age encampment, or in the court of a Stuart monarch, in the slums of nineteenth-century Manchester and in a modern hospital are different experiences which carry different meanings. A social meaning is one placed upon a label such as 'midwife' by a variety of social and public discourses and constructed by social policies. How can we 'understand' what it means to be a midwife in the last decade of the twentieth century ? Oral histories which record the remembered life experiences of midwives working in the past (Leap and Hunter, 1993) show vividly what this meant to individual women, but what does the occupational label of 'midwife' mean in society and how is it constantly reinforced in everyday practice? This is the object of our search.

The social meaning of a defined occupation is always in process, it is dynamic and ever-changing and can only be captured at a specific juncture as a snapshot captures a moment. This identity has to be constantly reinforced and reconstructed but must always retain a referral point of recognition for the practitioners to feel a sense of security in belonging. The ways in which an occupational identity is constructed and reinforced include work practices and strategies of control, use of language and public representations of this image. This is an essentially interpretive exercise involving the values and perceptions of the observer and the observed.

Recently sociologists have become very interested in the ways in which the professions of surgery and dentistry have constructed a social meaning (Fox, 1992; Nettleton, 1992). Midwifery is especially interesting to a sociologist not only because it is a gendered occupation but also because it operates in a private female sphere which has historically been shrouded in sexual mystery and societal taboos.

The social meaning of midwifery as an occupation cannot be divorced from the social meaning of childbirth, so the first step in this study is to look at the changing construction of the labour process itself. It is significant, we feel, that the very phrase 'labour process' is used to describe both the activity of childbirth and the organisation of work in an industrial economy.

The re-siting of birth from the private world of the home to the public world of hospital mirrors the change in the economic mode from private home-based handicrafts or agricultural work and small family-owned enterprises to large-scale factory production which has occurred since the advent of capitalist industrialisation.

The description of the hospital way of birth as resembling an assembly line is one which is often evoked by women and it is this comparison with an industrial organisation of labour which our study takes up.

A historical analysis of the changed role of the hospital midwife as the manager of the labour of others with the child as the object of production is set out in the first chapter. A wider understanding of the evolution of this role can be gained by looking at the specific identity of midwives as women working within this female sphere of production.

The hospital work practice takes place within a set of hierarchical and inter-professional relationships, therefore the second step in the exploration is to look at the strategies which midwives and the other professional groups such as obstetricians and GPs have employed in order to gain control of the labour process. When this theoretical background has been sketched in, the study itself will be presented in order to pose an interpretation of the ways in which all these themes come together in everyday life and work.

■ Studying midwives at work

The ethnographic studies which form the focus of this book were conducted in two British maternity hospitals during the latter part of 1989. The researcher was, and is, a midwife and undertook the research in her capacity as 'a student of research at the university'.

The two maternity units were quite typical examples of the provision of maternity services at that time and both formed part of the larger District General Hospitals. In 1989, as in subsequent years, 98 per cent of women gave birth to their babies in NHS hospitals (OPCS, 1991).

The usual practice was for women who thought they might be pregnant to consult their general practitioner (GP). The GP would write to the District General Hospital for an appointment for the woman to attend the booking clinic. This name derived from the time when a bed had to be 'booked' for the birth. The woman might see her GP again but more usually would next be seen at the antenatal clinic at the hospital. At this first visit the woman and her pregnancy would be assessed and arrangements would be made for 'shared care'. Shared care usually meant that the woman would visit her GP and then the hospital antenatal clinic on alternate occasions. Sometimes the woman would meet the midwife in her own home (another booking visit) or at the GP's surgery or health centre.

At the hospital it was usual to meet the antenatal clinic midwife and perhaps some student midwives. When the woman telephoned the hospital or just arrived, at the time of labour, it was likely that she would not have seen or spoken to the midwife before.

At the end of the 1980s midwives tended to stick fairly rigidly to 'their areas', i.e. the hospital antenatal clinic, the hospital labour ward, day duty or night duty. Generally only relatively junior midwives and students would rotate from one department to another and then only rarely to a community midwifery setting.

All the midwives in this study were employed by the Health Authorities and had a contract of employment to work either in hospital or in the community. All were salaried, some were part time (15–30 hours per week) and the rest worked full time at 37.5 hours per week. There were no temporary or bank staff employed and all were provided with uniforms, paid sick leave and thirty five days holidays per year.

■ The research

The research was conducted in two hospitals over a six month period during the winter and spring months. The hospitals were similar in design and in their state of repair and decoration although they were operated by two different health authorities.

Chapter 3 includes a detailed description of the methodology used for the study and considers the advantages and disadvantages of ethnography as a research method. It considers the ethical difficulties associated with the method and the issue of a midwife studying midwives.

The key themes that emerge from the study are presented in Chapters 4, 5, 6 and 7. Chapter 4 'Some aspects of labour ward culture' provides a detailed description of the setting of the hospital with the reader invited on a guided tour of the key areas where the observations took place. There is a detailed description of the multi functional 'office' with its unique features that formed part of one unit. There is also a description of the 'inner sanctum' or delivery room with an explanatory diagram. Further details of the environment are described with references to 'the notices' that formed such an important part of the delivery suite.

Chapter 5 is called 'All in a day's work' and considers the hospital admission procedure, the process of birth, and explores attitudes to blood and dirt. Admission in labour was observed to be a very routinised procedure where the midwife was seen to take control of the childbirth event. This control was clarified and confirmed during the birth of the baby, where the description includes the use of ritualistic phrases and expressions. The final section of this chapter considers the criteria adopted by midwives for the 'moral evaluation' of women and their partners.

In Chapter 6 (called 'Organisation and control') the reader is introduced, in the sections 'Getting through the work' and in 'Writing notes and drinking tea,' to the method employed by midwives to control the working environment. The study then considers the organisation of labour ward work including the control of admissions to the delivery suite, the dissemination of information and how the news of birth was spread. The use of terminology is explored especially the terms 'nigglers and labourers' where women were labelled according to the efficiency of the production process. This is further developed in 'Aspects of communication'.

Chapter 7 is called 'Shifts and handovers' and explores aspects of working shifts and the methods used to exchange information. It also studies other aspects of midwifery care. A typology of handovers is offered with analysis and comment. The difficulties associated with running a twenty-four-hour service are considered with attention being given to the unique features of night duty.

Chapter 8 reviews the key themes of Chapters 4, 5, 6 and 7 and debates the possible scenarios for midwifery care in the next decade.

The work of a midwife in the 1990s is inspiring, challenging, demanding, emotionally draining and absolutely unique. The study presented does not lay any claims for universality, it does not offer quick-fix answers for improving care. It aims to present information and analysis and seeks not to sit in judgement on the midwives at work in these hospitals. It is intended as a starting-point for analysis and constructive thought into the complex issues of care of women and their babies at a crucial time of their lives.

Chapter 1

The site of the labour process

The site of the labour process, as described in the study is that of a hospital labour ward, and this is, of course, the overwhelmingly common experience of birth for both 'labouring' women and practising midwives in Britain today.

Before we look at an example of the everyday culture of a labour ward as experienced and constructed by a group of midwives, it is essential that we place it within a comprehensible framework. For as a picture or a painting is shown to its best advantage when framed, so an ethnographic study must have a framework of historical and sociological explanation in order for it to be seen in full. This framework enables us to see the labour ward culture as something more than just an amusing account of 'a day in the life of a midwife'.

This labour ward culture must be placed within its social and historical frame, for it must be remembered that a study of midwives and mothers engaged in a normal birth in hospital would not even have been possible before the latter half of this century.

The purpose of ethnography is to show a familiar world from a different angle in order to make us question taken-for-granted assumptions and beliefs. In order to set the scene we must start by looking in more depth at the everyday common-sense knowledge that the hospital is the normal place of birth and the place for a normal birth, in Britain today.

The interaction between midwives, mothers and doctors takes place within a world bounded by the hospital building with its work organisation, rules, and traditions – a world which is known to many and therefore appears to require no explanation. But is this true ?

If we could put ourselves in the place of a person from another time or universe we would have to start by explaining why these women are in this place at this time and what importance society places upon their activity. If we adopt this identity of the cultural stranger to whom all must be explained, then the 'fact' of a labour ward culture emerging from the hospital setting cannot be taken for granted, it must be placed within its frame. It is important that this search for an explanation about the placing of birth be undertaken, as without it, it would be easy to fall into the trap of a one-sided and simplistic view which sees hospitalisation of birth as the one and only reason for the existence of some of the more controversial aspects of the labour ward culture which we shall describe.

We cannot begin to 'make sense' of this culture until we have an understanding of the changing meaning given to childbirth in our society, the site in which it takes place and the surrounding cultural and political climate within which the hospital came to be accepted by the majority as the appropriate place of birth in this society in the twentieth century. We have to answer the initial questions posed by the stranger: What is the status and meaning of childbirth and why is it taking place at this site?

Answers to these questions are essential if we are to begin to understand fully the labour ward culture which is described here, for when childbirth as an activity moved from the private female world of the home to the public masculinised world of hospital, it was a move of crucial historical and cultural importance. It was a move which overturned all previous historical experiences and set up completely new relationships between women themselves, created new professional practices and altered definitions of childbirth. The midwives who are engaged in the day-to-day occupational culture of the labour ward and the mothers who are admitted there are 'making sense' of this changed reality.

Before attempting to answer the questions on when and why this change occurred and its significance, let us consider the first explanation owed to the cultural stranger: what is the meaning given to birth in our culture ?

■ Childbirth, sex and motherhood

A pre-industrial culture which was more vulgar, earthy and open about sex and childbirth was replaced during the nineteenth century by the Victorian obsession with sexual appearance and behaviour and the rigid moral conventions imposed upon women.

An example of this cultural desire to cover up can be found in the practice of wrapping piano legs in cloth for fear that the sight of them would inflame desire, as well as the constricting clothes and corsetry within which women were enclosed. It is during this period that we also see the rigid division between the private and feminised world of the home and the public masculinised world of work being culturally and politically constructed (Hall, 1985; Davidoff and Hall, 1987).

However, ironically, the designation of all 'proper' female activity to the private world actually meant, in practice, that very rarely could women obtain any privacy within the home. Within the middle class Victorian household it was only men who were able to have a room of their own, a study, library or billiard room to which entry could be forbidden. Women's lives were more open to public scrutiny: if unmarried, they could not go unaccompanied anywhere and even if married with a 'home of their own', they had no personal space over which they had total jurisdiction. In the overcrowded slums and close-knit rural hovels, no form of privacy was possible but this meant that a cultural secrecy became even more important and although birth took place within the close proximity of both family and neighbours, it remained a secretive affair. Women often hid their pregnancy as if it were a shameful condition and it was never openly mentioned in mixed company. During childbirth women were often forced to refrain from crying out loud. In this cultural climate, childbirth was not a subject which could be discussed openly, it was a female discourse of pain, danger and secrecy.

Victorian prudery and salaciousness endowed pregnancy and childbirth with connotations of sexual sin. Within the social construction of femininity, based upon women as decorative, unsullied and passive, childbirth itself could not be defined as 'feminine'. The very act which proclaimed her identity as a 'natural' or 'real' woman was a taboo subject to be spoken of in whispers. Incorporated in the failure to confront the reality was the denial of the messiness, blood and pain of the experience. Male partners were nearly always excluded from attendance at childbirth, this was usually at the request of the mothers themselves (Humphries and Gordon, 1993) as well as orders by the midwife. Many of the later objections to the presence of the male partner at the birth were based upon the 'loss of mystery' and the undesirability of a man seeing a woman in an undignified and unrepressed situation.

For hundreds of years in cultural discourses from fairy tales to films, babies arrived magically, with the actual event of birth as an absence. In the world of high art following the Renaissance, the figure of the newly born Jesus was always depicted without an umbilical chord as if to deny the fact of birth. Even in popular films until the 1970s, childbirth invariably occurred off-stage and was accompanied by mysterious demands for hot water and the successful ending was signalled by the cry of the newly born baby. In recent years childbirth has been depicted on film but nearly always in the context of sex education or medical documentary.

More than a remnant of this puritanical attitude still exists today, for as recently as 1992 a nude photograph of a heavily pregnant Demi Moore on the cover of a magazine created great controversy, as did the famous Benetton advertisement featuring a bloodied newly born baby.

The great contradiction within this culture was that whilst romanticised pictures of motherhood flourished as a symbol of purity, the act of sex was regarded as polluting and childbirth itself was a taboo subject. Images of mother and child abounded in art and the figure of the patient and self-sacrificing mother was a common theme in literature and popular culture over the past centuries.

Childbirth, then, held a low status by its very absence from public discussion, and also because it was exclusively a female activity which was frequent and unremarkable. For most women, children were an inevitable part of their life, something over which they had no control. Until the nineteenth century children were not really regarded as beings in their own right at all. Sons may have been desired for dynastic purposes, 'to carry on the family name' or daughters sometimes 'for company' and 'to help in the house' or 'dress up' but children as such did not have a high societal value.

This view began to change in the late nineteenth century when the demands for labour power for Imperialist expansion overseas and industrial competition with other countries fuelled eugenic concerns over the quantity and quality of the population. The health and well-being of children began to occupy a central stage in developments in social policy, because of the need to produce factory workers and 'soldiers for the Empire' (Davin, 1978; Lewis 1980). As a result of these policies there occurred an expansion in the provision of maternal and child welfare services but the focus tended to be upon the healthy rearing of a child and not upon the childbearing process itself.

With the growth and extension of the state into all areas of family life, the child became a focus of governmental concern and responsibility throughout the twentieth century. Some of the cultural contradictions surrounding the act of childbirth and the status of motherhood remain in place, but the status of the child has changed dramatically. The pattern of smaller families and a decreasing birth rate has meant that children have become much valued and the centre of medical and health concerns. The infant mortality rate decreased at a far faster pace than the maternal mortality rate from the nineteenth to the early twentieth century.

The social meaning of childbirth has changed, from being a hidden event surrounded in female exclusivity and societal taboo it has become an open occasion attended by fathers and sometimes even grandparents, it has become a feature of home videos and popular TV and radio programmes. The taboos and hidden secret suffering which often surrounded childbirth in the past have been largely eradicated and it has been progressively sanitised, professionalised and mechanised. But as we shall see there still remains a 'private' enclave within which childbirth remains a site of female exclusivity and interaction even within the public domain of the hospital.

We now move on to address the next questions from the cultural stranger, when did this change of site take place and why?

■ Birth – from private to public

The resiting of childbirth which took place from the late nineteenth century and accelerated during the twentieth century mirrored economic and social change and fundamentally altered professional and popular images of childbirth and motherhood. Childbirth moved from the hidden all-female sphere, where the presence of men was taboo, into the open medicalised sphere where men were present and in control. This altered the social experience of childbirth for succeeding generations of women both as mothers and as midwives.

The growth in hospitalisation from the pre-war period in Britain to post-war was gradual but definable. In 1937, 35 per cent of all births took place in an institution and by 1944 this had increased to 45 per cent (Ministry of Health, 1949).

The hospital experience is now the norm but this is perhaps more recent than many suppose, as Figures 1.1, 1.2, 1.3 and 1.4 illustrate.

As can be seen, the period of greatest growth in the hospitalisation process was in the 1960s and 1970s, a period which saw the massive expansion in hospital-building programmes and changes in the organisational structure of the NHS.

The decades of the 1950s, 1960s and early 1970s were a period of economic growth and full employment which meant a labour shortage in some health occupations. Nursing, like other occupations, had recruitment difficulties and needed to offer inducements in order to attract staff. But the existence of more hospitals and the perception of the acquisition of a midwifery qualification as a good career move for the ambitious nurse, do not explain *why* hospital births had become the accepted and seemingly desired norm within a space of forty years.

Even though dissenting voices were beginning to be heard in the 1970s they were from a minority of mothers and midwives. By 1990, the period of our study, the almost total hospitalisation of birth had been completed. Both the midwives and mothers in the labour ward described here were of a generation which had been completely socialised into the normality of the hospital as the site of birth.

How and why had this happened ? In order to answer this question we must turn back to the pre-war period in order to trace the beginnings of this cultural change.

■ Making childbirth 'safe'

The initial moves by the State to remove childbirth from the private to the public sphere were conducted through political and medical discourses concerning infant and maternal mortality and the effects of these upon the birth rate. It was the maternal mortality rate which most concerned legislators on the practice of midwifery in the first half of this century. Midwives were seen to be responsible for the birth itself and its attendant and immediate dangers. Responsibility for both antenatal and post-natal care was a much later development.

Like much else in the founding of the post-war welfare state, the debates about the status of midwifery, of mothers, the provision of access to health care and of a more egalitarian childbirth experience, began in the crucial inter-war years. It was then that the debates on the relative merits of hospital and home as safe sites of childbirth and of the demarcation of responsibilities and areas of control of midwives and doctors became

Figure 1.1 Place of delivery in England and Wales, 1960

1960   800 824 births

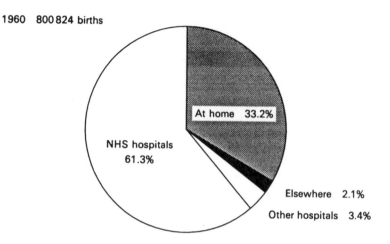

Source: Macfarlane and Mugford (1984).

Figure 1.2 Place of delivery in England and Wales, 1970

1970   794 831 births

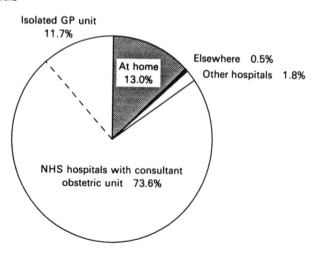

Source: Macfarlane and Mugford (1984).

Figure 1.3 Place of delivery in England and Wales, 1980

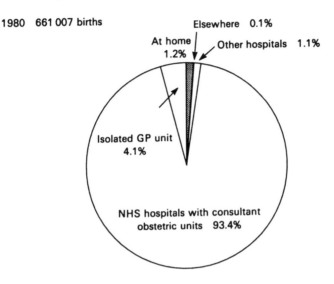

1980   661 007 births

Elsewhere   0.1%

At home
1.2%

Other hospitals   1.1%

Isolated GP unit
4.1%

NHS hospitals with consultant
obstetric units   93.4%

Source: Macfarlane and Mugford (1984).

Figure 1.4 Place of delivery in England and Wales, 1992

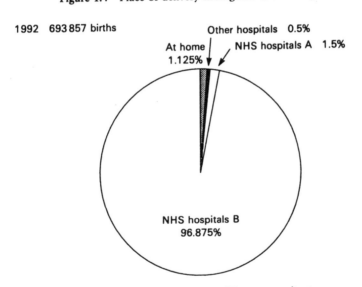

1992   693 857 births

Other hospitals   0.5%

At home
1.125%

NHS hospitals A   1.5%

NHS hospitals B
96.875%

A   NHS hospitals with beds allocated to GPs not consultants
B   NHS hospitals with consultant obstetric units which may have GP beds

Source: OPCS Birth Statistics (Series FM1, no 20) (London: HMSO).

public. These debates were conducted through the discourse of safety and the much publicised concern over the maternal mortality rate and falling birth rate during the latter half of the 1930s.

As in most other European countries, Britain's birth rate declined at this time and strange as it appears to us today, this was thought to be evidence of declining national power, confidence and prestige. The large loss of male lives in the First World War still dominated much public thinking and women were exhorted to have more babies. But it was feared that the relatively high rate of maternal mortality as well as the painful and debilitating experience of childbirth and its after-effects, could cause mothers to 'go on strike'.

Avoidable deaths from childbirth, the 'deep, dark and continuous stream of mortality' (Ministry of Health, 1937:51), had been a concern of the medical profession and the subject of governmental investigation from the 1920s.

In 1923, Dr Janet Campbell produced a report on midwifery training which included a section on maternal mortality in which she stated that antenatal supervision by a medical practitioner should be encouraged in order to cut the rate (Campbell, 1923:38). A year later in 1924, the first Government report specifically focused upon maternal mortality was produced – again by Dr Campbell. In this, she described both maternal mortality and morbidity as 'this burden of avoidable suffering' (Ministry of Health, 1924:5).

But it was the public airing of this network of concerns following the publication of increasing mortality figures after 1931 which acted as the engine for the change from home to hospital births. A detailed Government investigation in 1936 (Ministry of Health, 1937) had as its object the pinpointing of preventable deaths in named high-risk areas. Socio-environmental factors such as poverty, housing, unemployment, diet and even climate were considered but the Report failed to give precedence to any one overriding factor. What it showed were the clinical causes (see Table 1.1) and also the economic circumstances of the mother (see Table 1.2).

Two important factors emerge from a reading of this report: the significance given to clinical causes, and the inverse ratio of social class mortality. The higher maternal mortality rate among the better-off classes was attributed to the fact that they were more likely to have the services of a doctor than a midwife and to be in a private nursing home or maternity home which was more vulnerable to infection.

Surprisingly, the mortality rate (from puerperal fever) in affluent Hampstead was three times higher than in socially deprived Bermondsey (*News Chronicle*, 1934). It was reported in 1935 that in England the general lying-in death rate amongst better-off women attended by medical practitioners was 5 per 1000 which was twice that of midwives' patients (*Nursing Notes*, January 1936:2). This apparently greater rate of loss of

Table 1.1   Primary causes of death in childbirth

Class I: Deaths due primarily to child-bearing	Number of deaths	Percentage of puerperal deaths	Percentage of total deaths
(a) Toxaemia	137	21.31	17.79
(b) Haemorrhage	86	13.37	11.17
(c) Trauma	92	14.31	11.95
(d) Sepsis (not associated with abortion)	219	34.06	28.44
(e) Abortion	101	15.71	13.12
(f) Puerperal insanity (non-septic)	4	0.62	0.52
(g) Hydatidiform mole	3	0.46	0.39
(h) Unclassified	1	0.16	0.13
	643	100.00	83.51
Class II: **Deaths due to intercurrent disease**	127	–	16.49
	770	–	100.00

Source: Ministry of Health, Report on Maternal Mortality (1937).

Table 1.2   Economic circumstances of mothers who died in childbirth, 1937

Cause of death	Satisfactory (good and fair)	Poor	Very poor	Not stated	Totals
Toxaemia	92	37	4	4	137
Haemorrhage	49	33	–	4	86
Trauma	69	20	2	1	92
Sepsis	133	78	1	7	219
Abortion	58	39	–	4	101
Puerperal insanity	2	–	1	1	4
Hydatidiform mole	2	–	–	1	3
Unclassified	1	–	–	–	1
Death due primarily to intercurrent disease	58	61	5	3	127
Totals	464	268	13	25	770
Percentage	60.26	34.81	1.69	3.25	100.01

Source: Ministry of Health (1937).

middle-class lives therefore appeared to be due to their preference for the services of a doctor as opposed to a midwife. Why then did the middle classes appear to choose medical attention?

There was a minority who amid all the official pronouncements questioned the validity of the figures. For instance, a correspondent to *Nursing Notes* in 1934 argued that the apparent increase in mortality was in fact caused by the decreasing birth rate. (*Nursing Notes*, September

1934:139). In other words, as there were fewer babies being born then even an unchanged mortality rate would appear to have actually risen.

Another practising midwife noted that there was a larger number of first pregnancies which ended in death, because of the higher number of one-child families in existence especially among the middle classes. (*Nursing Notes*, September 1934:136).

There are of course, contemporary debates on the relative 'safety' of home and hospital with many writers arguing that home births were always, in fact, safer (Chamberlain, 1981; Ehrenreich and English, 1973). Nor were hospitals necessarily more hygienic, indeed Leap and Hunter (1993:12) reported that many midwives working in the 1930s remember hospitals closing down for 'drastic disinfection' following deaths from puerperal fever.

One explanation of the apparently higher rate of death in hospital as opposed to midwife deliveries at home was that the more problematic or 'abnormal' birth was much more likely to have been referred to a doctor and admitted into hospital. Therefore it could be argued, midwives and doctors occupied separate spheres of responsibility. The responsibility and indeed the skill of the midwife involved the ability to detect an abnormality and call for the services of a doctor. The definition of normal and abnormal birth thus became the organising principle around which the demarcation of medical and midwifery practice was to take place.

The widespread use of antibiotics and sulphonamides by the end of the 1930s drastically reduced the dangers of sepsis and was certainly the most important cause of the decrease in maternal mortality which accelerated after 1942. The decrease had in fact begun before 1939, so if the immediacy of the concern had passed before the beginning of the war, why did hospitalisation gain momentum?

As the report of 1937 had indicated there was no evidence to show that hospital as a delivery site was any safer than home, quite the reverse in fact. The debate over the relative safety of hospital and other sites including the home, is one which surfaced again in the 1970s (Tew, 1977) and is still heard.

■ Defining safety

But to concentrate on the rather vague term of 'safety' in this search for the reason for the acceptance of hospitalisation is to miss out a whole area of explanation. Whether a hospital was thought to be 'safer' by the majority of women is not really the issue, the point is, how was 'safety' defined? This is of crucial importance for us to understand, for we need to gain an overview of all the currents of ideas which were flowing around the important move to hospital which began at this time. These ideas were to dominate the female discourses about childbirth for subsequent generations of women.

Recorded views of women on the experiences of pregnancy and childbirth are relatively rare. The letters to the Women's Cooperative Guild (Davies, 1978) are a great revelation in this respect as they movingly describe the fear and dread with which childbirth was often viewed by women at the beginning of the century. Marjery Spring-Rice also recorded a similar picture of bad health, pain and deprivation among women in the 1930s. (Spring-Rice, 1939)

But probably the most common channel for the relating of childbirth experiences with which most girls became familiar at a young age, was by word of mouth. Tales of pregnancy and childbirth remained within a universal female subculture. Although the maternal mortality rate may have been a cause of public and political concern articulated by government and the medical profession, for most women death through childbirth was a very real possibility. But it was only that – a possibility – far more common was the acknowledgement that birth was painful and had long-term debilitating effects on health and well-being. 'Old wives tales' were exactly that, they were tales of personal experiences which were not pleasant but had a purchase on the truth.

Women of higher social classes sought to 'buy' for themselves a measure of relief and protection from the attendant dangers of childbirth, and as we have seen, this meant the attendance of a doctor. For even if they were not actually purchasing greater immunity from death, they perceived that a medicalised birth was in some sense more desirable. Why?

One reason was that the presence of a male undoubtedly added to the expectation of better quality of care even if this meant that the designation of potential abnormality was being made, but there was also another factor, which by the 1930s was gaining in public recognition – the relief from pain.

The perception began to grow that women themselves were adopting higher expectations and were rejecting the status of birth as a 'natural' phenomenon with all the connotations this phrase held. A striking indication of this growing trend is evidenced in the words of the government report of 1937:

> The increased sensibility to pain and discomfort has led to the movement to secure for women of all classes the relief from pain in childbirth which was formerly accepted as part of the course of nature (Ministry of Health, 1937:117).

This is an extraordinary statement in that it seems to imply that women themselves have changed and become more physically vulnerable to pain and also that this pain relief is not available to all social classes. This then is to be the next move to hospitalisation.

■ **Natural birth, pain relief and social equality**

As the official report of 1937 quoted above had noted, there was an increasing popular perception of hospital as the desired place for birth. Interestingly, what was emerging was a rejection of the 'naturalness' of birth and the posing of an idea of 'natural' birth against the desirability of a hospital birth. One correspondent to *Nursing Notes* in 1936 regretted this trend:

> You hit the nail on the head in your paper last week with the phrase 'Expectant mothers are hospital-minded' and incidentally exposed the root cause of our high maternal mortality rate. Childbirth is a natural function and not an illness, and if only we could bring our women back to this belief our death rate would drop to that of countries where babies still arrive in their own homes, or to that of our own midwives who work amongst the poorest mothers (*Nursing Notes*, June 1936:87).

This demand for increased access to hospital services remarked upon by her, was not a new one. As far back as 1915, one of the letters collected by the Women's Cooperative Guild had spoken of the need for 'a system of State Maternity Hospitals, where working women could go for a reasonable fee and be confined, and stay for convalescence' (Davies (ed.) 1978). Hospital therefore could be seen as a place to escape from the responsiblities and pressures of domestic life.

After the Local Government Act of 1929, many of the old Poor Law hospitals came under municipal control thus losing their stigmatising image. Before the advent of the Midwives Act in 1936, the cost of a hospital birth was refunded to people in the lower income groups, which frequently made it cheaper than the fee charged by private domiciliary midwives which was not refunded (Menzies, 1942:37). But as well as cost, there were other reasons why hospital was perceived as a desired alternative to the 'naturalness' of home.

It was as though it was the very 'unnatural' nature of a medicalised hospital birth which was increasingly being sought. What then could hospital and the medical profession offer which was the focus of this altered perception? It was, of course, the increasing availability of pain-relieving drugs and palliative techniques.

The control over the provision and use of these was to be one of the ways in which the medical profession effectively colonised birth within the precincts of the hospital in the years to follow. The medical profession through the Royal College of Obstetricians and Gynaecologists (RCOG) resisted any moves to allow midwives to administer chloroform whilst at the same time officially endorsing the extension of pain-relief to all women (RCOG, 1945). The social class inequity of access to pain relief was noted by the President of the Royal College of Midwives in 1934:

> One of the aims of civilisation was to prevent pain. For the final pains of
> labour the richer mothers had had chloroform but, as only a doctor
> could administer it, the poorer mothers were deprived of its help
> (*Nursing Notes*, 1934:93).

Although domiciliary midwives could use the gas-and-air Minnit machine
after 1936, the lack of transport and the sheer difficulty of carrying the
equipment mitigated against its widespread home use. But even though this
was a professional strategy which was used to further the interests of one
group as opposed to another, the demand from women for pain-relief was
very real and increasingly articulated.

The more 'natural' alternatives to pain-relieving drugs and medication
gained some publicity during the 1940s and 1950s, notably the more
'psychological' approach of relaxation as propounded by writers like
Grantley Dick-Read. But increasingly women were looking to the medical
profession and more 'scientific' solutions.

Material gathered by a Mass Observation (1945) study into the 'birth-
rate problem' and the reluctance of many women to have children
illustrates this point:

> I couldn't bear the thought of going through all that pain. I've just lost a
> sister in confinement and she was only 26, and a fine and healthy girl.
> She got buried with the baby, five weeks old. Well, it frightens me to
> death.

One letter from a doctor's postbag of the time read:

> I read in Reader's Digest some months ago of a painless childbirth which
> had been successfully introduced in America. An injection in the spine I
> believe. Why can't something of this kind be brought into this country
> and within the scope of all mothers?

Another commented,

> What is being done to make childbirth easier? Is anything being done?
> Or are all our brilliant doctors and specialists still content to tell us that
> childbirth is a natural function?

There is also evidence that many working-class women believed that a
pain-free childbirth was the experience of the wealthy and that they were
being denied this privilege. One respondent to Mass Observation study
said:

> The hospitals for poor people should be made as comfortable as the rich
> nursing homes are. Rich people don't suffer, why should we? They
> should make more beds available now. It's a real scandal these poor
> women not being able to get in anywhere.

Another:

> Yes, if you have the money you can have the best anaesthetics and everything. That's not right is it?

> I think science should do more for working people.

There is supporting evidence for this suspicion, a Government Report on Maternity in Great Britain in 1948 revealed that only 20 per cent of women having a home birth received analgesics compared with 52 per cent in hospitals and 77 per cent in private nursing homes. It was further revealed in the survey by the Royal Commission on Population and reported in a Eugenics Society meeting in 1947 that of those women confined at home three out of five from the professional class received analgesics whilst the figure for the manual working class was only one in five (*Nursing Notes*, February 1947:29). Therefore, greater access to pain relief and for some the relaxation of being away from home, made hospitalisation increasingly attractive to many women but until the foundation of the National Health Service (NHS) this was often not a realistic option.

We have briefly mentioned the professional strategies which were being used at this time, strategies of medical control over the administration of pain-relief and the definitions of 'abnormal' and 'normal' birth which were becoming more complex, and we will return to these in the next chapter. But some women at this stage of the upsurge in demand for hospitalisation had private reasons for not wanting a public hospital birth: the shame of poverty on the part of the working-class women and of social stigma on the part of middle-class women. Some of the reasons given by midwives working at this time can find an echo today. The poverty suffered by some working-class women made them reluctant to go into hospital as 'they hadn't got night clothes' (Leap and Hunter, 1993:141) and some were fearful of leaving husbands alone in the house. Many middle-class women also could not afford the high fees of a private nursing home and 'couldn't visualise themselves mixing in hospitals' (Leap and Hunter, 1993:141). We can see therefore that there were always some alternative sets of ideas which existed in parallel to what was rapidly becoming the dominant view.

We have argued that hospital was for many reasons, changing its identity as a site of birth. We finally need to investigate this in a little more depth: what expectations and beliefs about hospital birth have become common currency? In other words, what is the cultural reality which surrounds the interaction between midwives and mothers in the labour ward?

■ Popular culture and hospital

The expansion of the hospital service was one of the most significant changes which followed the foundation of the NHS in the post-war era.

This growth in the number of hospitals meant that for the first time in history admittance to a hospital became a common experience. Therefore the way in which people culturally defined a stay in hospital also changed dramatically. Historically hospitals had been 'associated with pauperism and death' (Granshaw and Porter 1990:1). But with the institution of the welfare state and the focus upon ideas of equality which were a feature of the post-war period, this identity underwent a transformation.

Like many aspects of social life in the post-war period, hospitalisation can be viewed as an example of a breaking down of class inequalities. With the NHS act of 1946 (implemented in 1948), equal access to health care at the point of need for all became a basic tenet of the post-war welfare state, and childbirth became increasingly seen as requiring expert medical attention to which all women were entitled.

The nationalisation of care for women in childbirth in the aftermath of the Second World War was the culmination of a process begun in the pre-war years. In a period of social reform and nationalisation of all public utilities the formation of a national maternity service fitted in with pre-war arguments and post-war emphasis on centralised planning. Hospital birth can be seen as an example of the egalitarian and modernising ethos of the years that followed, when home birth and midwives seemed to belong to a Victorian past and were connected with memories of poverty and deprivation.

This new way of birth reflected other aspects of women's lives. Everyday life became lived in a more 'public' and open manner during the 1950s, children went to school in large purpose built buildings, people went to work in 'open plan' offices or factory assembly lines, they lived in housing estates in identical modern houses with large open windows and the open aspect of the labour ward was only an extension of these.

At the same time, the popular representation of the medical profession was of a trustworthy miracle worker in a white coat. Doctors were almost beyond criticism and their authority unquestioned. Popular television programmes with enormous audiences reinforced this view. Programmes like *Dr Kildare*, *Ben Casey* and *Emergency Ward 10* presented this view of hospitals and doctors.

The 'normalisation' of hospital was achieved by the increasing exposure of the population not only to its building but also to its inherent values. The values of hygiene, professional expertise and control were carried into the private world of the home even before the actual process of birth was moved into the hospital.

When a woman had her baby at home the doctors and midwives concentrated on creating a mini-hospital in the home itself. Prospective mothers were shown how to 'prepare a room', to sterilise all necessary equipment and to adopt hospital techniques of hygiene which were in a sense, out of place at home. Everyday home life was disrupted by this and a clear distinction was drawn between 'normal' living behaviour and the new and appropriate behaviour required of responsible parents. Although very few births take place today in the home, this transfer of a hospital-like pattern of behaviour often takes place during post-natal visits. A community midwife or a health visitor will inspect the equipment bought for the baby and instruct 'parents' (nearly always only mothers) on the correct way to do things.

Conversely, within the hospital setting a 'home' atmosphere is created. Families and partners and other children may wander in and out at any time, photographs and cards are prominently displayed. The ward frequently contains children's drawings on the walls and 'thank you' cards to the staff from previous grateful occupants.

After the 1960s, as hospital births became the norm, this meant that many more educated middle-class women were recipients of a hospital-based system which did not allow for educational or social diversity or for individual desires and wishes. The collective provision of health care of which the maternity services were a part, were constructed for a homogeneous mass of pliant, submissive, 'grateful' and primarily working-class women who were content to take their allotted place in the line. During the 1960s and especially in the 1970s a generation of women emerged who had received access to further education, who were used to more freedom of expression than before and who, to a degree, were more self-confident. This change should not be exaggerated as it was only true of possibly a minority, but the general lessening of deference and the ability to demand consideration as an individual was a definable cultural attainment which had not existed before.

The reaction against the hospital way of birth emerged at this time and was coterminous with the growth and widening of feminism and a return to individualist values. In an era of political action and a reaction against science in many forms including nuclear power, the medicalisation and surgical interventionist techniques of control were perceived as the epitome of male scientific hegemony. The women who formed pressure groups such as the National Childbirth Trust (NCT) to campaign for more choice in the siting of childbirth and an extension of home births may have only represented an articulate educated minority (Reid, 1983), but it was a minority which was increasingly vocal and effective.

Within midwifery too, this reaction against hospitalisation of birth gained in support. The view of hospitalisation as an essentially retrograde step for both child bearing women and the work practice of midwives became voiced in most sociological and historical reviews and professional journals. This view can be summarised by a recent contributor to Midwives Information and Resource Service (MIDIRS) who demanded, 'How did we get into this mess in the first place?' (Cronk, 1992).

Throughout the 1980s these discontents became more widely expressed and the analogy of hospital birth as resembling a factory assembly line was almost a cliche.

But despite this growing opposition, hospital birth was the norm at the time of the labour ward culture described here and had been since the period when the midwives in the study had trained. So it can be seen that despite a minority of mothers who voiced their opposition and a growing occupational reaction against it, hospital as the place for birth was, and is still, the majority experience.

We have now completed our initial search for meaning, we have seen how the subject of childbirth has become more sanitised and open, placed as it is within the public sphere of the hospital. We have seen the part played by concerns over the danger of childbirth in the move of the site, and finally how and why hospitalisation became increasingly accepted even though in later years there have been objections from sections of the public and midwifery.

We have so far in the construction of our framework set out the background to the actual site of the working practice of the women engaged in the interaction of the labour ward. We now perhaps understand the meaning given to birth and the reasons why these mothers are here at this time. All the factors which historically brought women to hospital are still present: it is believed to be a 'safer' place, the provision of pain-relief is expected, medical control of the birth is unquestioned and the authoritative presence of a midwife automatically assumed. The 'naturalness' of childbirth has been in a sense rejected by the majority in the search for a feeling of security. The hospital, despite its connotations with illness and medicalisation appears to offer that security. Interestingly, the more 'natural' techniques of childbirth such as relaxation, breathing exercises and the water-birth have been incorporated into the hospital organisation. Increasingly, a 'natural' birth is being defined as an absence of any medical attention. A contributor to a recent series on the 'hospital and home' debate in a national newspaper summed up this attitude, 'Childbirth may be natural but it does not feel like that at the time' (*The Independent*, 1993). There may exist a resentment among mothers of some of the hospital rules or organisational practices, medical authority may not be quite so easily attained as in the past but they are here and they are subsumed into the site of the hospital for the duration of the labour process.

This part of the frame is now in place, it remains now to turn our attention to the person of the midwife in order that a total picture can be obtained.

Chapter 2

The management of labour

What exactly is a midwife and what are her function and status in the hospital process of birth? These are questions which a cultural stranger would ask and they need to be carefully considered. In order to do this, we have to throw away our common-sense assumptions and begin to look in more depth at the conventional and accepted position of the midwife.

The occupational identity of a midwife is the subject of this chapter. We have already seen that the site of her work was constructed by a network of external social policies, political philosophies, professional strategies, popular discourses and public demand.

A quick response to the question 'what is the status of a midwife and what is the meaning of her presence on the ward?' would be to reply immediately that she is a professional who has a clearly defined function in the management of childbirth.

Most practising midwives and many others would unequivocally claim that midwifery is a profession. The claim to a 'professional' identity is widespread, articulated and accepted by the majority of midwives, and each new cohort of students is socialised into this identity. But let us begin our questioning at this point, 'what do we mean by a profession?' and 'upon what basis is the claim that midwifery is a profession founded?'

■ Professions and semi-professions

What is a profession? Traditional sociology has defined certain occupations as professions by virtue of their claim to specific attributes. This 'trait' approach has set up requirements such as independence, autonomy, the possession of an academic education, a set body of knowledge, responsibility for practice, and the adherence to ethical standards. An occupation is assessed as a profession if it can be checked off against this list (Parsons, 1954; Wilensky, 1964). In this view professions were somehow seen as above political or personal prejudices and neutral and objective in their judgements. A strict demarcation line is drawn between a 'professional' judgement or action and a 'personal' one. A professional is to be trusted to give knowledge-based and objective decisions. The traditional professions such as law, medicine or the Church enjoyed a high status and prestige and received relatively high economic rewards throughout most of this century.

There were, however, always critics of this claim to objectivity and neutrality. Marxist sociologists would point to the upper- and middle-class domination of the professions and the neglected area of the concept of power which was absent from the dominant functionalist 'trait' approach. The question of power was placed in the centre of a revived sociological interest in professionalisation by Johnson (1972). He argued that a profession was not an occupation so much as an institutionalised means of controlling other occupations. This basically Marxist approach laid stress on the role of access to power structures and political interests within a specific historical period as the means by which professions gained the power to control others. It represented a demystifying of professional power as being related not to 'objective' criteria of expert knowledge or neutrality of intellect but to social power, class interest and political influence. This radical new approach opened up a new body of sociological thought which sought to analyse the meaning of professionalisation in our culture.

■ The professions: a man's world?

The increasing influence of feminist scholarship during the 1970s led to a further analysis of the social basis of the professions, for as well as being middle class the professions were seen also to be overwhelmingly male.

Historically, women's entry into the professions has taken two routes; either a few outstanding individual women gained entry to a previously exclusive male profession like law or medicine (and the Church of England in 1992) or a female-dominated occupation like nursing or midwifery sought professional status as a group.

Within sociology, these occupations have been placed under the heading of the semi-professions. Although still maintaining a basically checklist approach, this definition has placed gender in the analysis of a profession for the first time. Etzioni (1969) gave the initial classification of a semi-profession as an occupation which exists within a bureaucratic organisation and is staffed mainly by women. The presence of women meant, for Etzioni, that the desired characteristics of a true profession could not be achieved because of the inability of women to aspire to the attainment of objectivity, the exercise of authority and the tendency of women to engage in trivial discussions about personal matters (Simpson and Simpson, 1969). In short, as Anne Witz states, ' because women are not men, "semi-professions" are not professions' (Witz, 1992:60).

Ironically, the very qualities which are instrumental in the subordination of a feminised occupation such as midwifery, are thought by many engaged in midwifery education and practice to be its fundamental and core essence such as communication and empathy. But this poses a problem for midwifery as a female occupation aspiring to professional status: is it possible to erect an alternative system of values and attributes for the possession of a professional identity based upon a different set of criteria? The ethnographic study which follows illustrates that in the production process of birth, the end product (a live, healthy baby) has become the sole criterion of success with the actual process itself, the experience of labour and the interpersonal relationship between women and their carers being correspondingly marginalised.

If, therefore, professional values are masculine values and the semi-professions represent the subordinated 'female' area of practice, what exactly is their function and relationship to the dominant profession?

■ The semi-professions: a woman's world?

Jeff Hearn takes the debate a stage further when he maintains that the male-dominated professions only accomplish their work and maintain status through the functions of the female semi-professions. The main role for the semi-professions such as midwifery and nursing, he argues, is to take on the emotional labour involved in professional-client interaction. This absorption of the emotions thus enables the masculinised profession to avoid close personal contact and so maintain an 'affective neutrality' and objectivity which has already been constructed as the basis of true professionalism. A true professional can remain remote and in control because any threat to this state has been drawn away by the feminised semi-professions (Hearn, 1987:140).

The term 'masculinised' refers to the set of values and cultural assumptions inherent in the construction of the professional group and not to the gender composition of the group itself. Although there are female obstetricians (in 1994 there were 160 female Consultant Obstetricians which is 14 per cent) as there are male midwives (currently 0.1 per cent) this does not invalidate the argument that it is the profession itself as an entity which encapsulates the dominant value system.

Indeed many female medical professionals act in the established 'male' manner in order to gain professional credibility, as Wendy Savage so aptly describes (Savage, 1986).

A good example of this practice in a labour ward would be the emotional labour involved in comforting and coping with the pain and distress of a woman after a stillbirth. This task is most likely to be undertaken by a midwife who absorbs all the initial emotional bombardment before the doctor appears to sign the certificate. In this way professional power is reinforced through the subordination and non-recognition of this function of female labour power. 'People-work' such as midwifery, nursing, social work and counselling is thus seen as a 'natural' arena for the female qualities of caring, empathy and patience and so structurally these jobs remain female-dominated and of a lower status and prestige.

There is another important indicator of a lower-status occupation, and that is its visibility. Like any other occupation which contains an emphasis on 'hands-on' tasks or involves a close physical contact with a client group, the work of the midwife is very visible to others.

■ Power and distance

Michel Foucault (1977) argued that the development of organisational structures like prisons and hospitals had been for the purpose of surveillance of large numbers in an increasing population. The very design of these institutions constructed open spaces where many people could always be observed by the few, and so they felt permanently under scrutiny and adjusted their behaviour accordingly. In a sense they learnt to 'police themselves' because of the all-pervading observation by those in authority.

The design of Nightingale wards in hospitals was a perfect example of this analysis. The nurses' station was placed in the centre and those in higher positions of authority were placed further and further away from the visible centre (Kenny, 1993).

If we apply this argument to lower-status occupations we can see that this geographical and spatial analysis still operates all around us. The first people an outsider will see on entering any hospital ward will be a nurse usually of a lower rank; on entering a GP's surgery it will be the reception staff, and on the labour ward it will be a midwife. The holders of power, predominantly males, will be invisible; their authority will be present but they will be out of sight. The design of the labour ward in our study is evidence of this invisibility of power. The office is where midwives can escape from the public scrutiny and 'be themselves', where they can avoid the gaze of both the public (who are themselves being scrutinised) and the medical staff who are protected from surveillance because of their position of power.

Midwifery then occupies the classic terrain of the semi-professional or skilled worker but cannot be included in the definition of a profession. There is a circumscribed sphere within which a midwife may practise and this sphere has been constructed by another dominant profession. The power and autonomy of midwives working on the labour ward is fenced around by constraints which have been imposed historically and which are an everyday experience.

But the meaning of an occupation is a great deal more complex than just its definition as a profession, a semi-profession or a skilled craft. These labels communicate very little to the cultural stranger and will not enable us to understand the culture of the labour ward in any depth. What we need to ask therefore is: what does the category of 'midwife' signify and what is the nature of the relationship between midwives and other women?

■ The public image

Historically, the identity of the midwife as a woman dealing in the private and therefore 'mysterious' female world of birth has always occupied an ambiguous and contradictory cultural space. On the one hand, she was a skilled, knowledgeable and paid female worker and as such occupied an intrinsically different role from that of the woman giving birth, whilst on the other hand, the world in which she operated was a hidden one of taboo, male exclusion and ignorance. It was a world surrounded by rumour and superstition, within which the 'wise woman' occupied a position of limited power and authority.

It was, of course, this female possession of power which made her liable to charges of witchcraft and subversion in the Middle Ages and to charges of ignorance and backward practices in the nineteenth and early twentieth century.

Before the medicalisation and 'male take-over' of childbirth, the midwife may have occupied a specific place in the world of health care but it was always a subordinated one. As Mary Chamberlain has noted, 'Midwifery itself, because it dealt with women and was conducted by women, had low status' (Chamberlain 1981 : 25).

Because there was a low status accruing to all aspects of childbirth or indeed any activity which was performed by women, the likelihood of there being a 'lost golden age of midwifery' is remote.

Midwifery, by its very nature, took on the same cultural taboos that adhered to pregnancy and childbirth. As childbirth was absent from the popular and public culture so too was the depiction of the work of the midwife.

By contrast, images of nurses abounded in the public press, literature, history books and films. During the Victorian era and into the twentieth century up to the present, the romanticised picture of the nurse abounded. In times of war, the nurse was portrayed as the rather saintly 'lady with the lamp' caring for wounded soldiers. Other images of the nurse as a 'ministering angel' were part of a popular presentation of nursing. Interestingly, nurses were almost always shown with children or male patients but rarely with women. The other parallel image of the nurse was that of the sexy, young and rather flirty girl, an image which has continued from the *Punch cartoons* of the First World War to the 'Carry On' and 'Doctor in the House' films of the 1960s. Even today, a nurse's uniform is a fancy-dress symbol for sexual provocativeness in 'stripper-grams' and at college dances.

But midwives could not be co-opted into the same public image because their work concerned childbirth which was on the one hand a dangerous activity which often resulted in death, and on the other a female zone of hidden sexual connotations. One way out of this impasse was to present childbirth as a joke and so cartoons and photographs of the working midwife would show her as a 'nurse' presenting the proud father with a baby (or more likely twins or triplets) without the presence of the mother.

Interestingly, in language also, the address of 'midwife' does not exist. The most common form of address is 'nurse' and in pictures the midwife was always shown wearing a nurse's uniform. The other less-flattering representation of the midwife is one which was propounded by Victorian writers such as Dickens, that of a dirty, drunken old woman. This image is very powerful, and remained in the constructed image of midwifery until very recently. It was the background to demands by the medical profession that they be given the legitimate control of birth and to the aspiration to professional status by the newly-formed Midwives Institute. It was a portrayal which had to be eradicated by the attainment of public respectability.

■ The problem of respectability

The gaining of public respectability and acceptance was one of the motivating forces behind the aspiration to be identified as a 'professional' worker.

In a sense this was a problem for all women in the period of the emergence of more occupations which were visible to the public. In the nineteenth-century culture, women who went about in the streets and other public places were in a very ambiguous and potentially dangerous situation. During the latter half of the century women began to move out of the private sphere of the home and to be seen in the visible public arenas of the street, the school and the hospital. This move was surrounded by social ambiguity and danger. Judith Walkowitz has chronicled the ways in which many of these 'new women' presented themselves in order not to be judged as prostitutes (Walkowitz, 1993). Sexual harassment from 'male pests' was a deterrent for women, and for those working as nurses, charity visitors, sanitary inspectors and school-teachers, a personal identity had to be quickly established. This was one of the meanings behind the adoption of distinctive uniforms like those of the Nightingale nurses and of Salvation Army 'lasses'. These performed the function of badges of respectability for women who were operating in the unfamiliar territory of public spaces.

Midwives, however had different problems in establishing a professional and respectable identity. In a sense they had always operated in a semi-public sphere of work even if the nature of that work remained in the private sphere of the home. The sight of a midwife hurrying along a street at night did not necessarily excite comment or harassment, but it must be remembered that she was known and recognised by all in a small community. The urban working-class areas or even the rural villages where most midwives worked were very tightly-knit communities where she would have been recognised and known. Unlike women working in hospitals as nurses or in schools in unfamiliar territories, the midwife did not need to 'explain' her presence in the semi-public sphere of these communities. But the nature of her occupation remained a subject which was not publicly discussed. This local security of identity was not readily transferable either, as an anecdote in the Government Report on Midwifery in 1949 illustrated. This concerned a municipally employed midwife who was boarded in a small private hotel in a strange town during 1948. In this hotel she was requested not to use the public lounge as 'her presence might embarrass the other guests'! (Ministry of Health, 1949:2).

There was also another factor which made the construction of respectability especially problematic. Midwifery not only had to combat association with childbirth, it had also long been associated with abortion and procurement. The overwhelming majority of the women who were involved in these illegal activities would not have been registered or qualified but as far as the public was concerned they were loosely labelled and identified as 'midwives'. Chamberlain has argued, 'Where the working class were concerned, midwifery, abortion and the "still birth" business (infanticide) were one and the same in the public image' (Chamberlain, 1981:119). Midwifery had then to achieve certain specific characteristics in order to present itself as an occupational group aspiring to a higher status. For midwifery to engage upon this project, there had to be a radical transformation in perception, it meant that the old image had to be abandoned as well as a new one constructed.

A clear distinction had to be made in the public mind between the new professional and the old unqualified handy woman or 'woman you sent for', even if she also took the title of midwife. How was this to be achieved?

■ The road to respectability and status

This identity was to be constructed within midwifery by two connected routes; by the drive by the Royal College of Midwives to a publicly recognised status and by a change in the person of the midwife herself. Another important element in this construction was the change in the site of birth from the private sphere to the public hospital. But first a brief review of the steps undertaken within midwifery itself.

There are two crucially important dates in the project to gain status for midwifery, the Acts of 1902 and 1936.

The Registration of Midwives Act of 1902 was fought for by the Midwives Institute and a section of the medical profession. Its passage through parliament was a long one which was frequently delayed and bitterly contested. However, after 1902 a roll of those women who were considered bona fide (even if formally unqualified) midwives was constructed and published. This was an important development in two ways; first it eliminated from official recognition those who were considered undesirable, and it created a legitimate register. It brought midwifery out of the private enclosure into public view. Interestingly, one of the prerequisites for registration was, as is the situation even now, the necessity to be 'a woman of good character'. This emphasis on moral standards of behaviour was, of course, only applicable to occupations such as midwifery and nursing which recruited women. But this qualification signalled the move away from the past to a new public identity.

The creation of midwifery as a state-salaried service was completed in 1936 in the Midwives Act, against the background of the 'save the mothers' campaign. This move was overwhelmingly welcomed by the Midwives Institute and the press. The creation of a salaried domiciliary service offered the prospect of financial security and employment. This was an important factor as it was reported at this time that many independent midwives were facing poverty and hardship. Ellen Wilkinson, an Opposition Labour MP stated in the House of Commons during the ratification of the bill that as a result of the depression midwifery was almost a depressed trade with the majority not earning 'as much as £100 a year' (*Nursing Notes*, 1936:65).

The new identity of a salaried worker enabled the popular press to refer publicly to the work of midwives for the first time. The political campaign to reduce maternal mortality, of which the 1936 Act was seen to be a part, gained publicity particularly in the London County Council (LCC) local elections in 1937. For example, the *Daily Herald* carried the headline,

MOTHERS' SHOCK BRIGADE

The paper went on to report that '48 whole-time salaried midwives are to join London's shock brigade to fight maternal mortality' (*Daily Herald*, 1937:15). So it was that the fight against maternal mortality and the legislation concerning midwives were linked in the public discourse.

Within midwifery, the demand for qualifications had also grown with the century. From a basis of practical experience and good moral character, specific midwifery training became placed in the area of further training. Direct entry into midwifery declined and by the 1960s the midwifery certificate was regarded as the next step for the ambitious nurse.

It was sometimes viewed in the nature of a trophy which need not be used (only a proportion of qualified midwives ever practised) but one which the owner was proud to possess. It could therefore be viewed as not only an extension to nursing but as an added qualification. It could be said to be a badge of superiority, for after all it was not available to the more lowly-qualified nursing staff.

The change from the midwife as an untrained local woman with a dubious public image to that of a qualified and respectable practitioner was a journey which had taken many centuries. It also involved a different public presentation; in other words the person of the midwife underwent a change of image.

The most obvious way to signify a new respectable image was to change the appearance and person of the midwife herself. In the light of high maternal mortality, the accusation was often levelled at midwives that it was they who were the carriers of disease and they were often described, by doctors whose standards often left a lot to be desired, as 'polluters of the atmosphere' (Loudon, 1986). In the moves to sanitise birth, the midwife herself came to be sanitised.

It has recently been argued (Bashford, 1993) that the sanitarian discourse which emerged at the end of the nineteenth century and has dominated health care to the present time, required that the aspects of hygiene and cleanliness had not only to apply to buildings like hospitals and homes but also to the person of the health worker herself. Therefore, the old 'gamp' who was portrayed as dirty, alcoholic and sexually experienced had to change to the new 'professional' who was clean, sober, educated and unmarried although not too young. After all, unmarried and therefore 'pure' young women were not supposed to have knowledge of sex or childbirth and so the respectable midwife was expected to be of 'a certain age' even if she remained a spinster.

The newly-formed (1947) organisation of the Royal College of Midwives also personified the new professional approach and respectable appearance which was being constructed. A glance at the biographies of the founders of the Royal College (Cowell and Wainwright, 1981) show them to be without exception, educated, articulate, elegant and undoubtedly upper-middle-class ladies. They were women of strong character and determination who had dedicated themselves to a profession and in many ways personified the 'new woman' of the *fin de siècle*. Most remained unmarried and perhaps this gave them the social ability and freedom to negotiate with powerful medical men who could help the cause of midwives' registration. During this initial stage of the quest for professional status, one way in which midwives could navigate the complex network of male power structures was to become 'honorary' men! This often meant the suppression of any outward manifestation of vulnerable femininity or the responsibility for husband or children. This was the route taken by many newly independent women at this time in their attempt to open new paths of living and working in the public sphere and characterised a form of feminist identity which still remains today.

Many midwives, like other professionalising women 'gave up' a personal life which included marriage and children to pursue a vocation. This suppression of personal and private feelings often led to close living and working relationships between women. Walkowitz (1993) chronicles this pattern of 'spinster marriages' which were indicative of a feminist solution in the early part of this century. Interestingly it was the acquirement of a degree of public authority which gave these women a choice in their private lives.

The adoption of a masculinised approach to work and life was one way in which this new generation of professional women made sense of their ambiguous social position. In a very illuminating statement a midwife working in London during the Second World War stated:

> Then of course there were a lot of men away and we liked to think we were holding the fort for them, you know, looking after their wives . . . (Leap and Hunter, 1993:126).

But the necessity to be unmarried in order to pursue a career in public, diminished in the post-war world.

The demand for labour in the new National Health Service grew during these years, the marriage-bar operating against nurses working in hospitals was eliminated and the labour shortage of the affluent years of the 1960s and 1970s meant that there was a recruitment problem in nursing as in other occupations and consequently more married women entered into all spheres of paid work.

The public presentation of the occupation of midwifery had undergone an enormous transformation and it had gained in status and respect, but it had meant that it was not only that the old image had been shed in the transformation, but also the traditional sphere of work and the distinctiveness of midwifery practice.

■ Hospitalisation and the nursing connection

During the Second World War, midwives gained a more visible public presence when childbirth was included in the emergency services and hospitalisation increased and, concurrently, maternal mortality decreased. In 1944, the Royal College of Obstetricians and Gynaecologists (RCOG) proudly proclaimed that because of this increase there was now 'maternity accommodation in institutions for at least 50 per cent of the mothers of the country' (RCOG, 1944:25).

This process continued in the early post-war years with the creation of the national maternity service and the amalgamation of midwives into the hospital service.

Hospitalisation had a profound effect on the working practices and status of both obstetricians and midwives. The subordinated status which applied to childbirth was reflected in the low esteem with which even the male-dominated profession of obstetrics was regarded in Britain until after the war. The Royal College of Obstetricians and Gynaecologists was not formed until 1929 and this formation was achieved against great opposition from the traditional enclaves of the Royal Colleges of Surgeons and Physicians. It did not achieve royal status until after the Second World War. It is obvious that the process of hospitalisation created a space for the professional grouping of obstetricians to gain in power and status. Indeed, many writers argue that the move was prompted solely by the professional ambitions of this group but conducted within the discourse of 'safety', but as we have argued, the definition of this was riddled with contradictions. But, as has been argued in the previous chapter, the reasons behind the move were a great deal more complex than just the achievement of the professional ambitions of one group. What was the impact on midwives and their practice and status?

The hospital domination of midwifery practice continued unabated in all the years following 1948. This was to have a great effect both within midwifery between the two divisions and between midwifery and nursing.

In the immediate post-war period, domiciliary midwifery services continued, for as we have seen the great increase in hospital births did not occur until the 1970s. But although the midwifery services were divided officially into two sections of district and hospital midwifery, the 'independent' midwife had ceased to exist after the 1936 Act. Domiciliary midwives were employed by Local Authorities and increasingly took on antenatal and post-natal work which the newly NHS-contracted GPs no longer needed to do. This pattern continued with the emphasis on antenatal services increasing as birth itself was removed from the 'community' to the hospital. The majority of qualified midwives were based in hospital practice by the 1970s and this took on the appearance of the 'normal' realm of midwifery work. After the NHS reorganisation in 1974, the integration of hospital and district midwifery meant that the district work came under the control of the hospital service, thus ending the formal division between the two sections within midwifery itself.

Midwifery had always insisted upon an independent identity and on the formal separation from a connection with nursing. The two occupations had historically had different colleges and organisations but within the hospital setting, this division had became less obvious. Both wore starched uniforms and both were addressed as 'nurse' by the public and both were working under the face-to-face control of the distanced medical profession.

The problem of creating a completely separate identity became even greater after 1978 when, in implementing the Briggs Report, the state officially sanctioned the amalgamation of midwives, nurses and health visitors. This move was vigorously opposed by many, especially those who were arguing for a more radical approach to the creation of a specific identity and work practice of the midwife. In 1983 the interests of midwifery and nursing were amalgamated in the creation of one central national statutory body, the United Kingdom Central Council for Nursing, Midwifery and Health Visiting (UKCC) and four national boards of nursing, midwifery and health visiting for England, Northen Ireland, Scotland and Wales. Within these moves the identity of midwifery was perceived by many to be in danger of being completely submerged into nursing.

With the official movement of amalgamation into hospital services and its formal connection with nursing, it became even more important for midwifery to draw around itself an identifying line. The move into hospital with the public sanitising of childbirth, had in some respects, enhanced the status of midwifery. It had become a good career option for the ambitious nurse and it had given a measure of security of employment. But for the identity of midwifery as a separate and definable occupation, this new site of working was problematic. How could a definable division be drawn between midwifery and nursing with whom it was now so closely linked? The very proximity and close relationship between the two made the restatement of midwifery's 'special status' even more important. As externally the two occupations came to resemble each other, so the necessity to be perceived as different became paramount. But upon what basis could this identity be proclaimed?

■ The idea of independence

The concept of independence as applied to actual practice and to the occupation as a whole is the primary distinguishing characteristic of midwifery. A glance through any midwifery journal or conversation with any group of midwives will illustrate how much the identity of the 'independent practitioner' is accepted as a basic and fundamental criterion of midwifery practice. Each generation is socialised into the abiding concept of the midwife as an independent autonomous practitioner. As this is such an important reference point for an occupational identity, it is crucial to attempt an 'unpacking' of this concept which is so often taken for granted.

It is the application of the idea of an independence in working practice which ideologically sets apart the occupations of nursing and midwifery. Midwifery has staked a claim to a degree of superiority to nursing in this respect. The annoyance and indignation which follows if a midwife is referred to as a nurse by the uninitiated, will bear witness to this claim, not only of difference but of superiority. In order to clarify this ideological divide, a conceptual map needs to be drawn so that a clear picture of the perceived differences between the two can be portrayed. This map is as follows:

Midwifery	*Nursing*
Independent practitioner	Dependent 'handmaiden'
Partnership with doctor	Subservient to doctor
Manager of normal labour	Carer for the sick
Health	Illness

It is, of course, a matter of debate as to whether these ideological categories can be justified in reality or in actual practice. Many nurses would perhaps take issue with the typology of the subservient nature of nursing but nevertheless I would argue that these do represent generalised categories of concepts which, however crude, most would recognise and acknowledge to some degree. Recent ethnographic studies of nursing have, in fact shown that the deferential attitude of nurses towards doctors can take many forms (Porter, 1991; Hughes, 1988).

It is the claimed status of independence and managerial control which sets midwifery apart from the bulk of nursing practice in the hospital site. This cloak of independence and autonomy is wrapped around the recruits into midwifery. After all, to achieve this status nurses had to undertake further qualifications and now there is a direct entry to midwifery for suitable candidates which by-passes any exposure to nursing practice.

In all other respects midwives are subject to the same organisational rules of pay and employment in hospital, and as Jean Walker (1976) has noted, the site of the work practice remained the same for the qualified midwife as it had been when she was a nurse.

In the past decade of the 1980s, nursing too has made great efforts to 'professionalise' itself, with an involvement in higher education, laying stress on research and a managerial presence. Nurses as 'managers of care' is an image which has gained currency with the changes in nursing education.

Midwifery however, has a longer history as a separate and identifiable occupation and, I would argue, took the 'managerial' identity throughout the hospitalisation process in order to retain an aura of independence as practitioners. What did midwives manage? The answer, as always, was the process of 'normal' birth, but this process itself changed and became an event dominated by the application of technology and intrusive techniques. By the 1970s then, it had gained an image of technological expertise, and although this may now be thought of as a retrograde step, it was not perceived as such at the time. Association with high technology made midwifery look scientific and progressive and a very far cry from the sepia image of the 'woman you sent for' at home. The command of the technology belonged to the dominant profession of obstetrics but midwives formed a strata of technical experts able to translate and apply technical orders from above. In other words, they became a perfect example of technical and process management. The actual production process of birth had been revolutionised and the relations of production had changed accordingly.

This new role for midwifery has been criticised by many writers (Oakley, 1984; Towler and Bramall, 1986) who saw this as a downgrading of role from that of independent practitioner to the status of an obstetric nurse, although other writers (Dingwall *et al.*, 1991:171) argue that to define this as a dilution of their role is misleading and that midwifery has become re-skilled rather than deskilled (see our argument in Chapter 8).

But if the claim to a management role can be substantiated by midwifery, why then the insistence on the possession of something called 'independence'? Is it merely a word which is used to distinguish it from nursing? Is it a legacy from the distant past when a degree of independence of action and self-employment was held?

Whatever the answers to these questions, it will be seen from our study that the adherence to a belief in independence of action is a very real one.

In order for the cultural stranger to really 'understand' the labour ward culture this background to the ideas which inform action and behaviour must be clearly drawn. The claims to independence and the assumption of a managerial role are carried into the labour ward as part of their equipment by the working midwives. But there remains one more area to examine before we can complete our framing of the picture, and that is the nature of the relationship between the two sets of women, the mothers and the midwives.

■ Professional power and authority

The two concepts of power and authority are frequently confused in everyday language and description. But I would argue that sociologically they can be distinguished and it is important to understand the different nature of the two when looking at the wielding of female professional power.

Max Weber gave the classic definition of power and of authority as a legitimated form of power. He argued that power can be simply coercive, as exercised by physical threat or social and emotional blackmail. He wrote:

> In general we understand by power the chance of a *man* or of a number of *men* (my emphasis) to realize their own will in a communal action even against the resistance of others who are participating in the action (Weber, in Gerth and Mills, 1970:180).

Authority however, is based upon true and 'freely' given consent. Others obey not because of fear, but because of a genuine and unquestioning deference to and acceptance of a greater authority. The relationship between the professional and the client has historically been based upon the claim to legitimate authority. The basis of legitimacy, for Weber, is characterised by three forms:

- it is rooted in tradition,
- an appeal by a political demagogue,
- by legal rational means,

This last form is the basis of professional power:

> [There is] domination by virtue of 'legality', by virtue of the belief in the validity of legal statute and functional 'competence' based on rationally created rules (Gerth and Mills, 1970:79).

People 'obey doctor's orders' or 'take professional advice' simply because of this acceptance of authority based upon expertise, experience and superior knowledge. In this and other situations such as that of the military, it is not the individual person who is laying claim to this position but the person as representative of professional authority. It is only in this one specific area that the person has this claim, once outside it the authority disappears. This position of authority is often signified by the wearing of certain clothes, like judges' wigs and gowns, surgeons' masks, doctors' white coats, which symbolise the professional not personal authority.

But as we have seen the professions which claimed this legitimacy were historically exclusively male, and so this authority appeared as a 'natural' male possession which was, of course rooted in tradition as well as claiming legal validity. This leads to a series of questions regarding women and authority: is it possible for women to transcend their gender identity and claim legitimated authority? Or will they always be perceived as women first and foremost?

■ Female power and authority

For midwives, as for other female workers in occupations which involve the exercise of authority, the relationship between their personal identity as women and their official 'face' is problematic. Traditionally, there has only been one area wherein women can possess a degree of legitimated authority – that of motherhood.

Within working-class and ethnic cultures there has always been an acknowledgement of a sphere of female power. This sphere was in the home over specific areas of life and within family and kinship networks. The existence of a cultural heritage of traditional 'mother-in-law' and 'Jewish mother' jokes bears witness to this recognition. But even within these communities, and especially within working-class cultures, this power of the mother is limited to the home and family which is the only area of traditional legitimated female authority. But even within this there are gradations of mother power within cultures from the London matriarchs described by Willmott and Young (1960) and portrayed in *East Enders* and *Coronation Street* to the classic Welsh 'mam' or Italian 'mamma' but it tends to be private power and not transferred into public authority. Mothers may have power over their own family but not as of right over other families or children. It is not to be confused with universally accepted authority. This point was made by Janet Finch in her explanation for the failure of self-help playgroups in working-class areas (Finch, 1984).

Within their own home this power is also often curtailed especially within a household with a male partner in residence; areas such as children, food, choice of furniture and decor, or perhaps holidays are designated for mother power, but the limits of her power as mother are bounded by the front door.

In many ways it is an area of power and influence which itself defines and limits any other area into which women may move. Women are crucially defined by their family relationships. Even women of prominent power 'in a man's world' are defined as 'mother' or 'wife'. One has only to remember the way in which Margaret Thatcher was portrayed as cooking her husband's breakfast in Number 10! The Queen is portrayed as a worried mother, and the Princess of Wales as a disappointed wife, in the popular press.

The exercising of power and authority outside this sphere is therefore always problematic.

Women working in the masculinised professions such as medicine, may possess a claim to a position of skilled expertise but they are still primarily regarded by others as women. The concept of 'professional power' cannot be claimed by women in the same way as it can be attributable to men. It has been argued that male professionals from an ethnic minority face similar problems in imposing an identity of authority (Hughes, 1988; Porter, 1993). An essential part of the identity of a professional is dedication to one sphere of activity coupled with an acquired knowledge and expertise. This does not necessarily include any element of personal experience or empathetic relationship, in fact in many ways, as we have seen, it is in direct contrast. Male professionals claim an authority in areas where personal experience is impossible (for example, obstetrics) but this does not mitigate against their perceived expertise. The majority of childbirth and child-rearing gurus have been male but as detached professionals they can claim an abstracted intellectual expertise in these matters. Women who more closely resemble this male detachment and single-minded dedication appear to 'fit' the definition of a professional. The implication underlying both a formal marriage bar and the assumed right to enquire into women's family arrangements is the assumption that a 'family woman' cannot be a serious or a 'real' professional as her duty is primarily to her family. Unmarried or childless women may approximate more closely to the ideal type of professional but they are also placed in an ambiguous position as women.

If the exercise of power is problematic for those women who are accepted in the masculinised professions, for women working in these areas and especially in the 'semi-professions' like midwifery or health visiting, the picture is more complicated and contradictory.

How are they perceived by the women who as mothers form their clientele? Many childless midwives or health visitors have been faced with the spoken challenge to their authority of 'How many kids have you had then?'

In the face of this charge many are forced to pose a form of acquired intellectually based expertise as the basis for their professional authority, but have they succeeded in one area only to be defeated in another? In other words, can a female 'professionally' based authority prevail over the traditional and 'natural' female authority of the mother?

Female workers as women have had to extend the range of female limited home-based power into the public sphere. Historically, there has been a series of strategies to circumscribe and set limits to this power. In the changing world of the late nineteenth century, women began to move into the new occupations such as health visiting, nursing, factory inspection, housing management and teaching. As the role of the State became more interventionist in these years, many middle-class women created a greater social and occupational space for themselves in these areas. But the concerns of public health, housing and education although receiving more state attention were still within the female orbit of influence. Women's roles in these areas were circumscribed by the male authority of the State and the medical profession but individual women workers were allotted a wider sphere of authority which did impinge in the public sphere. Over whom was this authority to be exercised and where?

Within public health, the authority of the new female occupations was still firmly limited to the private world of the home and especially the working-class home. Davies (1988) has shown how the gender division was drawn between the male work of health inspection which was placed in factories and slaughterhouses and the female work which concentrated on sanitary conditions of private homes. Women could not, and were not allowed to, have authority over men. Even female factory inspectors could only report on the working conditions of female employees. Health visiting was founded on the idea of 'educating mothers' and of the individualised home visit which meant that her authority often superseded that of mother power but she was not required to confront the male authority of the father (Davin, 1978; Symonds, 1991).

Within elementary school teaching, women took charge of infants and younger children or girls but rarely, if ever, older boys. Nursing was a female caste which was presided over by the individual female authority figure of the matron who had power over the nurses and a degree of restricted power over male medical students but the real authority was, of course, vested in the dominant medical profession. Eva Garmonikow (1984) has illustrated how this power relationship in hospitals between doctors and nurses closely followed the pattern within the patriarchal family with doctor as the father figure, nurse as mother and the patient as child. But even if it was curtailed and limited this was a new model of female power which was now being publicly exercised.

Where did midwives stand in this scenario? After 1906 they too were recognised as qualified and legitimated workers. They moved out of the hidden and private world of childbirth into a public role in health-care provision. But they were specifically 'different' from the other female occupations. Neither power or authority was a new phenomenon for midwives, they represented a recent organisation but not a new occupation for women. They had a purchase on a form of traditional authority which was not the case with other female professions. In the histories of early midwifery practice it is difficult to locate precisely the status of the midwife compared with her clientele. But increasingly her practice became concentrated among a poorer section of the working-class as the more affluent opted for the services of the higher-status doctor and the facilities of the private nursing home. Within this subordinated world of the working-class home the midwife undoubtedly occupied a position of authority which was unique. She alone could exercise an authority over the husband or partner of her clients in a way which no other female occupation achieved. This included the ability to exclude them from their own social space in the home. As one woman interviewed by Leap and Hunter reported: 'I think she was more for women than men, you know. She just dismissed the men as OUT' (Leap and Hunter, 1993:20).

This authority, however, was not a constant, it could only operate within the actual event of childbirth and not beyond. Also, of course, this was still the traditional female sphere from which non-professional medical men had always been excluded. This unique position placed the midwife in a complicated and contradictory set of power relationships with labouring women, 'ignorant' men and expert professional medical men.

How then can we understand the exercising of authority within this network of relationships in the sphere of the hospital? Midwifery is of course bounded, and its sphere of practice defined, by the dominant medical profession. The only thing that differentiates its position from that of nursing is the presentation and adherence to the concept of independence. But structurally, the medical profession has historically

deli
neg
V
res]
pro
son
defi
cha
esp
pov
T
hos]
con
mid
and
mas

[Handwritten annotations overlaying text:] Authority based upon expertise, experience + superior knowledge. Assembly line process, there is a constant flow, the emphasis is on the speedy - successful delivery of the product. laborers (mothers) → production area (ward) → product (the child) → line manager (midwife) final authority of the ward manager (consultant)

factors which underlie behaviour patterns and occupational cultures. These factors such as the creation of a separate identity for midwifery, the projection of an image of independence and autonomy and the need by an occupational group to claim a status of professionally-based knowledge and practice, all mitigate against any radically different alternative.

■ Completing the frame

We began by stressing the importance of a frame for the picture of the ethnographic study of the labour ward culture. This frame is now complete. In these two chapters we have attempted to illustrate the structural and cultural factors which have placed these women in this place at this time.

The structural factors described have ranged from the examination of some of the motivations which lay behind the move of childbirth from the private sphere of the home to the public world of the hospital. Social policies which prompted and accelerated this move were based upon a set of political imperatives which were centred upon the equal treatment of all social classes and the acceptance of the perceived demand for medical attendance and supervision of childbirth. The hospital became the 'normal' place of birth and not, as it was initially, the place for 'abnormal' birth.

This move changed the cultural placing of childbirth itself. By medicalising this 'natural' event, hospitalisation gave childbirth a public recognition that it had lacked. In a sense, the defining of it as potentially 'unnatural' and placing it within the medical and scientific orbit upgraded its status. From being an event which was surrounded in mystery and dread it became a subject for open discussion which took place in a hospital ward. Childbirth took on a different set of meanings and became the focus of technical intervention and scientific application. This was a cultural as well as a structural change in the experience of childbirth for the following generations of women.

This change also had an effect on the occupational status of midwifery which also took on a different set of meanings. As Garmonikow likened the working relationships in the Victorian hospital to that of the familiar authority patterns of the patriarchal family, we would argue that it is more useful to liken the labour ward relationships to those of the Fordist production line. Within this, midwives manage the labour of others. The site of the labour process is often likened by women to that of the factory assembly line, and in many ways this is a very apt description. As in the assembly-line process, there is constant flow, the emphasis is on the speedy and successful delivery of the product. In this case we have all the main actors in place; the labourers (mothers), the production area (labour ward), the product (the child), the line manager (midwife) and the final authority of the works manager (consultant). The midwife is in control of the day-to-day production line and only needs to get external support from the consultant when that line exhibits anomalies.

The debate as to the professional status of midwifery is not an intellectual game but is of crucial importance in reconciling the occupational ideology with real-life experience. The hospital practice of midwifery fulfils the function of a feminised semi-profession which is bounded and dominated by the masculinised profession of medicine. This is an everyday lived experience of hospital midwives. Independence and autonomy may have a strong ideological influence on midwifery, but in everyday practice they have to be constantly redefined.

The antagonisms and conflicts which are present in interaction between midwives and others stem from the contradictions of the ideological and the lived conditions of work. The exercise of power and authority is one area within which these conflicts emerge.

This structural and cultural framework is essential for an 'understanding' of the labour ward culture for without it, as Porter has stated, we could just take an ethnographic portrait as unproblematic and as 'speaking for itself':

> By ignoring the possible constraining nature of social structures, commentators are in danger of giving consent, through silence, to their oppressive effects (Porter, 1993:596).

The midwives in the study do speak for themselves in words and actions but it must be remembered that in order to 'understand' and not just communicate elements of this culture it must be framed by its structures.

Chapter 3

Ethnography: treating the familiar as strange

■ Studying the social world in its natural state

Ethnography is a very special type of research method that is particularly suited to the complex task of studying health professionals at work. As Kirkham (1992) has so clearly described it is a method used to study the social world of midwifery in its natural state, as it happens and where and as it is.

Dingwall (1992) argues that social research is a precondition of modern democracy. He says:

> It is only by the systematic study of our social existence, of how we live, where we have come from and what possible varieties of human social organisation might be that we can make available to all citizens, directly or indirectly, the knowledge that makes informed choices in social or economic policy possible (1992, p. 172).

He goes on to say that there will always be a place for the quantitative study of social behaviour and that some questions will arise naturally in the quantitative form of 'How many? How much? How often?' But others, he believes are intrinsically qualitative and ask the questions: 'For what reason? In what manner? How justly?' Such questions, Dingwall believes require answers from rigorously designed and dispassionately executed studies such as this ethnography.

There is very little that is straightforward about the work of a midwife in a hospital labour ward. Other research methods may focus on one small aspect of care whereas ethnography offers a broader approach. It aims to discover the unpredictable, the unknown and the unexpected. A questionnaire is frequently restricted to the researcher's sometimes limited agenda and may reflect only some of the issues, whilst a survey is likely to produce standardised responses from midwives who feel they are required to offer the current perceived wisdom.

Ethnography on the other hand involves having no preconceived ideas, it requires the researcher to look carefully, watch what happens and ask what various actions might really mean. It asks what makes individuals do what they do, it asks why they do what they do, and when they do it.

Ethnography requires careful thoughtful analysis and the meticulous follow up of complex problems. It is only by examining a culture in all its richness, intensity, colour, taste and volume that new facets of midwifery can be uncovered, described and given serious thought and consideration.

To those working in midwifery, life on the labour ward is all-consuming, there is little time or energy left to step back and consider the complexity of events and interactions. There is even less time to consider what it all might mean and why midwives do some of the things that they do. Ethnography provides that opportunity, the chance to consider in great detail minute aspects of being a midwife.

There is much disagreement in the sociological literature as to the precise definition of ethnography and how it differs from all other qualitative research methods. Hammersley and Atkinson (1983) describe how the key distinctive features of ethnography vary according to the perspective of the author. Spradley (1980) sees ethnography as the elicitation of cultural knowledge; while Gumperz (1981) describes it as the detailed investigation of patterns of social interactions; Lutz (1981) describes holistic analysis of societies whilst Walker (1981) explains it as an essentially descriptive technique presented as a form of story-telling.

There is also much confusion between ethnography and what Glaser and Strauss (1967) have called 'grounded theory'. Grounded theory is the development and testing of theories, hunches and ideas that may explain reality but that emerge from or are grounded in the data collected during the study. Some authors (e.g. Field and Morse, 1985) argue that grounded theory is a form of ethnographic data analysis and unlike phenomenology assumes the existence of a process. The constructs and concepts described are grounded in the data and the hypotheses that are 'induced' are tested as they arise in research.

Spradley (1979), whose name is often linked with the ethnographic method, describes how unstructured ethnographic interviews, which provide one type of data, can be analysed. Hammersley and Atkinson (1983) state that ethnography is a research method which draws on a wide range of sources of information or uses multiple methods of data-gathering. They say the ethnographer:

> participates, overtly or covertly in people's daily lives for an extended period of time, watching what happens, listening to what is said, asking questions; in fact collecting whatever data are available to throw light on the issues with which he or she is concerned.

It is a complex, detailed, meticulous research method.

There has been a much-publicised long-running battle between those who favour quantitative or positivist research and those who adopt what is described as a naturalist approach. On a simple level the positivist argues that if it cannot be counted, it does not count, whilst many qualitative researchers fall into the trap of trying to overcompensate for the effect the researcher may have on the data.

Hammersley and Atkinson argue that an ethnographer cannot escape the social world in order to study it, nor is it necessary. They argue that the researcher must inevitably avoid relying on a 'common-sense' knowledge and cannot avoid having an effect on the social phenomena being studied.

This discussion does not aim to present a defence of ethnography nor to counter the arguments presented by positivists – it does not need to. The views expressed by Hammersley and Atkinson (1983), Borhek and Curtis (1975) and Hammersley (1983) are that the first and most important step towards resolving this conflict is to recognise the reflexive character of social research and accept that we are all part of the social world we study. This research did not try to eliminate the effects of being a midwife doing research in a hospital labour ward but tried to understand what those effects might be.

Many of the criticisms of this type of study are associated with the role of the researcher as non-participant observer, some even argue that it is only when the researcher becomes participant that rich data can emerge (Leininger, 1969). These criticisms ignore the progress away from the 'fly on the wall' or full participation to the stage when the researcher becomes an active participant in the research process. The aim in this study was to maximise the benefits of being human and a midwife with sometimes inconsistent and unstable behaviour and attitudes and then to explore in depth the role of the researcher in shaping the context of the research. The key feature in this stance is the internalisation of the concept of reflexivity (Hammersley and Atkinson, 1983:14–23). This requires the researcher to accept whatever knowledge he or she has and treat it as valid in its own terms. It accepts that the researcher is part of the social world s/he studies. In this research the ethnographer was a midwife of some considerable experience and as a teacher of midwifery it was not surprising that the writer brought to the study knowledge of the field and some firm opinions as to what constituted good practice.

In this study there was certainly difficulty and anxiety associated with the prospect of developing the ability to treat the familiar (a hospital labour ward, albeit an unfamiliar one) as 'anthropologically strange'. The search for meanings in circumstances and situations that were familiar was very difficult at first but not impossible. As Dingwall (1992) states: 'Empathy has its place in ethnography but it should enter after recording rather than being confused with it.'

Ethnography makes use of basic skills such as listening, watching, asking questions and the skills of 'sussing out'; these are the self-same skills that anyone uses when, as a stranger, they try to make sense of any new situation. Ethnographers are part of the social world they study but they are able to develop the ability to stand back and reflect upon themselves and the activities of that world. This is *reflexivity*.

Ethnography is not in competition with other research methods but it is clearly a method where the advantages have previously been under-estimated. It is a flexible adaptable method which can change direction and allow the researcher to follow up leads and hunches, even change focus if this seems appropriate. As a method it is unique in that it studies activities, processes and interactions *in the context in which they take place* and not in artificial situations constructed for the purpose. It uses a variety of different information sources and thus allows data to be systematically compared.

■ Researching continuity of care

As explained, ethnographic research does not have a clearly predetermined research design but is a process that responds and develops throughout the period of the study. All research begins with some areas of interest or with particular problems to be addressed and ethnography is no different. When the research was being planned (1988/89) one of the key areas of concern in midwifery was the organisation of the maternity services. The move to almost 100 per cent hospital birth had resulted in a system of care where women and their partners would meet many different midwives during the childbirth experience.

The reports and enquiries which led to the current pattern of maternity care are reviewed in the Health Committee Report (1992). The key issue at that time and indeed later in 1992/93 was that of continuity of care and of carer. Indeed the Health Committee Report (1992) concluded:

> There is a strong desire among women for the provision of continuity of care and carer throughout pregnancy and childbirth, and that the majority of them regard midwives as the group best placed and equipped to provide this.

The key pressure groups for women were as active in 1988/89 as they are today. The National Childbirth Trust, the Maternity Alliance, the Association for the Improvement in Maternity Services, the Stillbirth and Neonatal Death Society were all campaigning for an improvement in the organisation of maternity services that would reduce the fragmented care available to most women.

Flint and Poulengeris (1987) in a report of a randomised controlled trial described how care could be improved by organising midwives into teams.

In 1987 the idea of totally changing the way in which the maternity services were organised seemed almost an impossibility. Indeed it was not until 1992 that the Government ordered the Health Committee to produce a second report into the maternity services. This report was followed by the setting-up of a Task Force whose report *Changing Childbirth – Report of Expert Maternity Group* and recommendations were published in August 1993. These reports built on the demands for changes and improved continuity that began as early as 1980.

In 1988, when this research was planned the view was taken that while there was probably a place for some midwives to work in small teams as described by Flint and Poulengeris (1987), the more urgent need was to try to improve on the existing arrangements for care. In particular there was felt to be an urgent need to minimise the adverse effects of discontinuity of care.

The disruption in the care of women in labour was most acute when one midwife went off duty and handed over the care to another midwife; a situation that never, or rarely, occurred in home birth or in the days of the lay midwife. One of the major areas of interest at the start of the study was the shift handover. Using a variety of ethnographic techniques such as listening, watching and asking questions, reading records and notes it was proposed to consider in detail what happened when the midwives changed shifts. I wanted to know what happened, where it happened, who said what to whom, who said nothing, how it was said, how it was reported and how it was recorded. I also wanted to know what midwives thought about the handover process. The aim was to look carefully at the social meaning and cultural actions that formed this social action. I was interested in all aspects of the midwives' work and especially in the culturally embedded norms that guided the action of these midwives.

The aim in this pre-field-work phase was to turn the so-called 'Foreshadowed problems' (Malinowski, 1922:8–9) – in this case concern about continuity of care – into questions that the research might be able to answer. The question simply was: could care of women and their babies be improved in any way at all?

■ Getting started

It was decided that the fieldwork for this study should be conducted in two maternity units which were fairly close to my home. Frequent visits were anticipated and the constraints of time and cost were considered. It was thought that two units in different health authorities but within reasonable travelling distance would be the best solution. I had worked in most of the maternity units in Health Authority A, so sought access in Health Authorities I have called B and C where the maternity units were new to me. Health Authority C responded positively to a simple letter written to the Chief Administrative Nursing Officer. Hospital B proved to be more difficult. Initially I made an informal approach to the Director of Midwifery Services, who listened carefully and asked me to put my request into writing. The response indicated that I should informally approach the following staff: the Senior Midwife, the Director of Nursing Services, the

Unit General Manager, the Chief Area Nursing Officer, the three obstetric consultants, the Committee Chairman of the Division of Obstetrics and Gynaecology, the Senior Midwifery Teacher, the District General Manager's secretary and perhaps the Health Authority Ethics Committee. This process took around six months. Each person I met wanted an explanation of ethnography. Most were unhappy with the research proposal I had prepared because, for example, 'details of the questionnaire to be used were not included'. Another respondent asked for clarification of the control group whilst a third wanted more details of the statistical tests that would be used. The medical team listened carefully to my explanation of the methodology and rephrased the proposal as some 'psychological research about communication'. It seemed easier to accept their interpretation of ethnography and thus expedite the start of the study, rather than argue.

The ethics committee wrote and asked if the Division of Obstetrics and Gynaecology were satisfied with the proposal. When I wrote back and explained their interpretation of ethnography and subsequent acceptance of the proposal, the ethics committee also gave its consent, with no conditions attached. After nearly nine months I had the official permission of all the gate-keepers in this health service hierarchy. This was despite the fact that I was a registered nurse, registered midwife and bound by the requirements of the UKCC Code of Professional Conduct.

I have no doubt that the interpersonal skills acquired over twenty or so years in health care were an important factor in obtaining access. However despite the fact that formal access was granted, negotiation with the 'gate-keepers' of each shift, on each visit, was also necessary. This was more of a difficulty in the early days of the study when there were more people who did not know what I was doing than did. It is also important to note that access is more than officially gaining entry and the right to observe admission procedures, care in labour and birth, but was renegotiated with the woman, her partner and the midwife on each occasion. Access to documentation such as medical and midwifery notes, the record book, the delivery-suite birth register, the off-duty books, the drugs book, the ordering book, the message book and even the duty request book had to be separately negotiated each time.

Throughout the process of negotiating access I carefully explained that I would not put women and the families at any risk whether physical, emotional, spiritual or psychological. I would always respect their rights of privacy and confidentiality.

■ **Choosing the site**

As described in the previous section it was thought to be important to consider the activities of midwives in two hospitals. Other factors were that I wanted to look at midwifery and midwives in an area where I was unknown (although this did not turn out to be the case) and where access was possible. The two units, in different health authorities, were probably quite typical of maternity units in the UK at that time. This view is confirmed by reference to the study conducted by Garcia and Garforth (1989) which described labour and delivery routines in English Consultant Maternity Units.

These findings also confirmed the results of a national study into the role of the midwife in the UK (Robinson *et al.*, 1983). In Garforth and Garcia's (1987) study 'Admitting – A Weakness or a Strength' similarities between the care offered by midwives in those units and the care in The Valley Maternity Unit can be seen. The Valley Maternity Unit as such does not exist. The descriptions and observations are based on information obtained from two hospitals in Health Authorities B and C. Some minor details of both maternity units have thus been changed and interchanged so as to protect the anonymity of the units.

■ Sampling

A series of thirty or so visits in total were made to either or both units during the winter of 1989 and the spring of 1990. The visits were initially arranged so that observations could take place at all times during the day and the night. Each shift change was considered in detail and involved observation at 7a.m., 2p.m. and 9p.m. In addition numerous visits were made to follow up the themes that were developing. Visits were conducted on different days of the week and at different times of the day and the night. Sometimes the visits lasted some eight or nine hours, sometimes only two or three hours. In the early stages of the study the temptation to stay all day and all night in order to see and hear everything was very strong but the first attempt to produce field notes after a thirteen-hour observation period soon convinced me that shorter periods of observation were more sensible and manageable.

In the initial stages there was a plan to include some unstructured interviews in order to examine and explore specific topics with key staff. I had anticipated that 'key' staff would be the midwives in charge of each shift. In reality the key informants included the most junior midwives, some student midwives, the 'nursing auxiliary' in one unit and a group of women who had their babies and who sat in the hospital day room.

These interviews were unstructured but carefully planned and deliberately probing. The analysis followed the guidance offered by Spradley (1979, 1980) and by Lofland and Lofland (1984).

■ The fieldwork stage

□ What can a researcher wear?

This is the story of the fieldwork. It began when I arrived at the maternity unit and went first to the Senior Midwife's office. She greeted me warmly and said she had explained to the Sister on the labour ward that I had been a midwife, but was now a student at the University. She explained that I was doing a type of psychological research on communication in labour. We went to the labour ward where she introduced me.

The Sister-in-charge explained that her son was at University studying psychology and offered me tea. I accepted and sat in the office with two midwives and an 'auxiliary nurse'; the labour ward seemed quiet, there were no doctors and only occasionally a student would walk into the office. The Sisters chatted and I explained that I was interested in looking at all aspects of the labour ward. They seemed happy to help. I explained that I would also ask each woman and her partner for their consent before observing them or aspects of their care. I chose to wear a skirt, blouse and a white coat in the first instance. This seemed appropriate and seemed to satisfy the senior midwife and the labour ward Sister. It was unusual for anyone other than the woman and her partner to be on the labour ward without a uniform. There was some concern expressed by the senior midwife that in ordinary clothes I might be considered a 'relative' and by implication an outsider and thus denied access. It was also thought that if I wore a midwife's uniform I would be expected to take responsibility for care. The white coat and its symbol of medical supremacy proved to be a passport to all areas. During the total fieldwork stage I was only challenged once as to my identity and position. One person said 'You are medical, aren't you?' as she ushered me into the delivery unit. This was more of a statement than a question and I said I would explain later. For someone in a white coat it appeared that access was unrestricted. There was little evidence of an awareness of the security risk or indeed the potential danger to women and babies. At a later stage in the study all staff were issued with identification tags complete with photographs. As the research progressed I abandoned the white coat as I believed it represented a dishonest assumption. Ordinary clothes became generally acceptable. They resulted in the medical staff almost always ignoring me. One female doctor asked which University I was at but that was all. I was initially a non-participant observer and spent my time watching as carefully as possible all that happened. I asked a lot of questions and listened to what was being said, by whom and to whom on every possible occasion. I became skilled at obtaining clarification and confirmation. I learnt the technique of noting what was not said and who chose not to contribute to discussions and conversations. I avoided carrying a brief-case and a clipboard and restricted myself to a pocket sized spiral note book and a small hand-held dictaphone. I spoke to most of the staff on duty on each occasion. All were willing to talk and answer my questions and even the most reticent would talk freely whilst cleaning equipment or making up beds. Without exception all the midwives and other staff spoke openly and freely to me in response to my questions. The atmosphere in these 'off stage' areas, usually during the period after the baby was born, appeared relaxed and I was openly included in the conversations.

In the early days of the fieldwork I divided my time between the office, the sluice room and the delivery suite. I used my standard introduction whenever I met anyone new to me, i.e. 'Hello, I am a midwife studying part-time at the University. I am looking carefully at the work on the labour ward to try to understand it more'. I felt like a newly appointed staff midwife, everyone was friendly, but I was unsure of where I fitted in. The activities I observed were familiar, but I wanted to be more comfortable in the environment. Something deep in my background told me I would be more acceptable if I was useful so I began by helping to change the soiled linen and refuse bags. It seemed to work, the staff accepted me as the study progressed and offered complete freedom and access to all kinds of information.

■ Participant or observer?

The maternity unit was frequently very busy and the staff seemed happy to cast me in the role of someone who was an additional pair of hands with some inquisitive and quirky habits (note-taking, etc.). During the early fieldwork stages (the first two or three weeks) it was clear that the staff were making a very special effort to be good communicators. One midwife asked if I would tape her as she encouraged or coached a woman in the second stage of labour. It was an outstanding, energetic performance, worthy of its tape-recording and the language will be familiar to many midwives. The midwife gave the woman instructions as shown in Field note (FN) 3.1.

FN 3.1

'Take a deep breath in, now hold it, now push as hard as you can, push push push, down into your bottom – not into your throat. Quickly take another breath, push push push, keep it coming keep it coming, push push push, don't waste the pain. Okay, rest a while!'

This was repeated verbatim during each contraction as the second stage progressed. The performance seemed to call for an applause and the midwife smiled and seemed almost to bow at the end. She asked if that was what my research was all about. She explained she thought she was a good communicator and I should put this in my research. I promised I would. This hyperactivity and desire to please and demonstrate communication skills lasted only a few visits. The staff quickly adapted to my presence, relaxed and began to act in a way that I recognised as being more 'normal', or at least not a special performance.

Ethnography aims to tell the story as it was, sometimes the result sounds rather patronising or even unfair but the researcher must record what he or she sees as honestly and accurately as possible.

My aim in this study was to be an observer but as one who was able to participate in such a way as to produce a relaxed feeling about my presence. The staff knew I was a midwife and in this respect this allowed me to move from complete observer to sometime-participant. This proved to be the most successful mode, it enabled me to become more and more reflective about the social world I was studying. Total participant observation, overt or covert, perhaps as an employed midwife, was practically and financially impossible. Hammersley and Atkinson (1983) argue that throughout the fieldwork the ethnographer must be 'intellectually poised between 'familiarity' and 'strangeness' while socially he or she is poised between 'stranger' and 'friend' (Powdermaker, 1966; Everhart, 1977). He or she is, in the title of the collection edited by Freilich (1970) a 'marginal native'. This describes my position in both of the maternity units of this study. I was on the outside and on the inside at the same time, and never really 'at home'.

■ Collecting, recording and thinking about the data

The maternity units in both hospitals consisted of an antenatal ward, a delivery suite, offices, an admission room, sluice rooms and storage cupboards, etc. Both units had a special-care baby unit and post-natal wards where women would be taken to recover from the birth of the baby. In this study only the areas sometimes known in both hospitals as 'the delivery suite' were included. This area included the office, the admission/ treatment rooms, a small four-bedded ward, the delivery room and the cleaning and sluice rooms. The practice in both hospitals was to call these areas the 'labour wards'.

My data collection took a variety of forms. The main activity was the production of field notes. During the visit I would use my notebook to record headings and key phrases that would help me in the recording. I also used the dictaphone, usually in the toilet or store cupboard, to record key phrases and prompts. After each visit, when I returned home, I would write detailed field notes on the events of that visit. These were initially filed in date order. The field notes would include details of events and accounts of conversations. Much of the time was spent observing and informally interviewing those who had emerged as key informants. These interviews were unstructured and in the early days I recorded as much as possible of what was said, how it was said, to whom and on what occasions. The field notes also include lengthy descriptions of the labour ward, the office, the admission room, etc. The staff were eager to help and went to great lengths to explain to me 'how it was', working in the delivery suite. Simple questions would result in complex and lengthy responses from all staff.

I practised and developed the technique of ethnographic interviewing as described by Spradley (1979). I interviewed individuals as and when the opportunity arose. I did not decide the questions in advance but knew the areas I wished to discuss or clarify. These areas nearly always emerged after I had written up the field notes following the previous visit. There were areas that were unclear, or where I had chosen to delve further into a specific aspect. The questions would be open-ended and would often lead into new areas. The field notes were generally descriptive accounts of events observed in the field. Direct quotations were included whenever possible as were descriptions of such aspects as the tone of voice and the body language of the contributor. The field notes also included sketches of some aspects of the environment and maps to remind me of the layout of the unit. Noting the position of doors and windows proved to be particularly helpful. During the research I was allowed unrestricted access to a variety of official and unofficial documentation. I made use of these sources to check data and to enhance the cultural picture of life on the labour ward. I looked at the midwifery and medical records, the Kardex, the birth register, the message book, letters from women and their partners and the notice boards. Learning what was appropriate to record in the field notes was important. After a few visits I realised that three hours observation tended to result in up to nine hours note-writing. The analysis was becoming more and more daunting. Spradley (1980) suggests a checklist that can be used to guide the researcher in the making of field notes. The checklist is as follows:

Space	physical place or places
Actors	the people involved
Activity	set of related acts that people do
Objects	the physical things that are present
Acts	single actions that people do
Event	a set of related activities that people carry out
Time	the sequencing that takes place over time
Goals	the things people are trying to accomplish
Feelings	the emotions felt and expressed

(Spradley, 1980)

The checklist proved to be a useful guide, as at quite an early stage there was the danger of being submerged in the data generated. Interviews were recorded separately, some were tape-recorded and transcribed whilst others were recorded from memory as soon as possible after the visit.

The second most important feature of the data-collection stage was the fieldwork diary. This was used after each visit to record my thoughts and feelings after each visit. From this diary emerged the type of questions that I felt needed to be answered. This was a most important stage in the theory-building phase of the study.

I also made use of what Hammersley and Atkinson (1983) describe as the analytical memo. I used a red pen to write notes and comments in the field notes. These notes were the early thoughts on the analytical process. They summarised my review of the field notes and subsequent reflections. Sometimes the notes were subsequently unhelpful, such as 'What did she mean by that?' or more helpful – 'seems another aspect of gaining control'. This was an important exercise and part of the process of reflexivity: the aim was to prevent me from returning to my natural mode of midwife. These analytical memos provided the signposts for the first stage of analysis. Themes were already beginning to emerge and aspects that required further clarification and explanation were revealed.

Hammersley and Atkinson (1983) argue that data recording is necessarily selective and involves some editing. It is true that the field notes for this study reflected the initial interests in shift handovers and aspects which 'caught my eye'. I aimed throughout the study to improve and build upon my reflexivity. I tried to observe and collect data on what was happening rather than look for incidences and examples to support my own biases and preconceived notions. The results can be judged in the findings.

■ Ethical and other problems

I was aware from a very early stage of the study that the validity of the research was threatened by my own occupation. I had chosen these hospitals because I had not worked at either and they were both within reasonable travelling distance of my home. What I did not anticipate was finding that I knew many of the midwives. For some years prior to the study I had been the 'Obstetric Nurse Teacher' at the local training hospital. Student nurses undertaking the compulsory twelve-week maternity care module had been taught by me. In three years some 300 or so students had completed the module and a significant number had gone on to become midwives. The hospitals in the surrounding areas now employed these women as midwives.

I was anxious that my role as a midwife and former teacher should not be confused with my role as essentially a non-participant observer. This proved to be very difficult on some occasions. It would be ridiculous to suggest that the scene being observed would not have been altered by my presence, but I believed that this effect reduced over time. I felt more and more that I was observing the 'real world' and not one constructed for my benefit. The situation was also altered by my unintentional participation as a midwife. I found it almost impossible not to talk to women and their partners. I have no doubt that on occasions my presence and contribution must have inhibited or changed the interaction between the midwives and the women. On the other hand it could be argued that my interaction was not very much different from that of the midwives so could be said to blend in with 'normal' events and communication patterns on the labour ward.

Hammersley and Atkinson (1983) warn:

> Even in the case of unsolicited accounts one can never be sure that the presence of the researcher was not an important influence. Even when the researcher is not a party to the interaction but simply in ear-shot, knowledge of his or her presence may have a significant effect (1983: 111).

This effect cannot be avoided in any type of ethnographic research. The midwives knew that I was a midwife and had in the past been a teacher. They seemed reassured to know that at the time of the study I was a student, or 'stay-at-home mother' and only working as a midwife part-time. This lower status increased my acceptability. When I met a different midwife it was not uncommon for them to confirm my status by saying 'You are not a teacher now then?'

It is true that I experienced difficulty in separating professional judgement from ethnographic work. My supervisor would refer to the 'Hunt Crusading Zeal' as I focused on aspects of care that I considered inappropriate or falling below my own high standards.

In the early stages of the fieldwork this aspect clouded my judgement and impaired my objectivity. I improved upon this weakness by creating a category in my field notes for 'angry thoughts'. I was able to take instances of poor or just-good-enough practice and label the offending aspects. Once filed under appropriate headings, I was able to take a more detached view and begin to understand what was happening and ask why I was feeling angry.

It was at this stage that I created my own model of midwifery care. I adopted the Rogers (1983) model of 'Unconditional Positive Regard' as a description of the relationship between midwife and woman. It was when I saw midwives who did not appear to share this philosophy that I became angry and frustrated. The model extends to the basis of the relationship that should exist between midwives and midwives. If midwives really have unconditional positive regard for each other they cannot help but work in a supportive and caring way.

■ Midwife and researcher

As the study progressed I became more reflexive and was able to view this particular social world more and more as an ethnographer and less and less as a midwife. I was beginning to be able to use my established knowledge and skills to understand this world more clearly. There were other dilemmas that arose 'in the field', apart from talking to women. Talking to women was not really a dilemma, but, as explained, that intervention was bound to alter in some way the scene I was trying to observe and of which I was simultaneously a part.

At an early stage I had to decide whether to answer the telephone. It rang very frequently. On a busy unit any help was appreciated and I was certainly able to answer the telephone and deal with most routine enquiries. If I answered the telephone there was a danger that whilst involved with dealing with the call, I would miss out on key issues I was trying to note and observe. On the other hand it was clear that letting the phone ring and ring would irritate, if not alienate, the staff of this busy labour ward. Despite this I generally chose the latter option, if I was in the room and no one else was available I would answer the telephone and try to pass on the question as quickly as possible. There was a danger in slipping into the role of receptionist and whilst the office provided a good vantage point I did not feel I was capable of being a full-time ethnographer and full-time telephonist. My view would be limited to the office. There were, however, more serious issues which challenged me in my role as a midwife-turned-researcher. My Field note 3.2 tells the story.

┌─ FN 3.2 ──────────────────────────────

Today I was in the delivery suite with S/N B. Mrs J. was in labour and the notes indicated that there was a breech presentation. The second stage was approaching and the midwife showed no sign of calling an anaesthetist, obstetrician or paediatrician to be on stand-by for the birth. I wondered if I should interfere. Perhaps she had telephoned and warned them without my knowing. Perhaps they were on their way. There were some signs of fetal distress. I wondered If I should suggest she telephone for help.

I didn't. The baby was born and needed resuscitation. An anaesthetist was called for the retained placenta. The post-delivery debate was acrimonious. Why had this midwife not summoned medical aid? The medical staff cast about for the person who would carry the blame. I must ask 'Why had this researcher not been interviewed?'

After this incident, where fortunately the baby and the woman were alright, I decided that in future I would always intervene if there was a risk to mother or baby. This was not as easy as I had hoped. On another occasion I was in the delivery room with a woman, her partner and a student midwife. Labour appeared to be progressing well although I noted some early deceleration of the fetal heart rate on the monitor. The door of the labour ward opened abruptly and a midwifery Sister looked in and stared at the monitor. She said 'Oh God, she's dipping' and the door slammed behind her without further comment. The student looked anxious, the woman alarmed and her partner distressed. If I intervened, the relationships between the woman and the midwife, and the midwife and the student would have been undermined. I took the risk and explained to woman, partner and student that there was no cause for alarm. In my opinion the alteration in the fetal heart trace was associated with the approaching second stage of labour. The woman looked appreciative and said 'Thank you, Doctor'. I had, of course, previously asked her permission to be present and had explained my status. The temptation to comment, advise and participate remained great but as the fieldwork progressed I became more proficient at dealing with it.

Fieldwork as a method of gathering data places the researcher at greater risk of encountering moral and ethical problems. Field research is at the sharp end and the ethnographer is not usually shielded from unsatisfactory incidences. The researcher is exposed to all aspects of the environment, the good and the bad. As the fieldwork progressed I became aware that a relationship of trust and even camaraderie had developed between me and the staff of the labour ward. I felt I was viewed more as a friend than an outsider and gradually took on the role of a sympathetic listener, even though I was on the outside and the inside at the same time. As this trust grew I was allowed more liberal access and invited to observe events from which I would have previously been excluded. I was encouraged to share in the birth of a stillborn baby and co-counselled a student midwife for whom this was her first experience of death in midwifery. The qualified midwife was concerned with supporting the woman and her partner but the student was left alone to fend for herself. As these relationships developed it became more and more clear that I should respect that which was told to me in confidence. I knew that I had a moral obligation to protect the rights, interests and sensitivities of those I was observing. It was crucial that I always acted in such a way as to safeguard and promote the interests of individual patients and clients (UKCC, 1992). To refuse to act or intervene so as to protect the research setting was morally indefensible. Research should never have a greater value than the value of individual women, their partners and their experience of childbirth.

To summarise, one of the main difficulties of this study was the task of separating professional judgement from ethnographic analysis. My considerable translation competence, or the in-built ability to translate or understand issues in midwifery practice, was a factor of which I had to be continually aware.

■ Analysis of the data

The analysis of the ethnographic data actually began in the pre-fieldwork phase when the research problems both topical and generic were identified. Topical problems were those considered to relate to the particular type of social setting, in this case the problems of offering and providing continuity of care and carer to women in labour. Generic problems relate to features of many different types of settings or people, which in this case were the aspects of controlling the work process.

In the fieldwork section I have already described the writing of analytical memos which were statements of ideas and hunches that guided the analytical process. It will be noted that this study did not begin with very specific hypotheses prior to the fieldwork but these were generated in the course of the study. The aim of this ethnography was to generate theory where possible and to identify the social processes that were occurring in this setting.

The analysis of the data was part of the research design and the subsequent data-collection was linked and led by the developing theory. In this study the observation led the researcher to hypothesise that there was a link between the quality of the shift handover and the stage of labour. Subsequent field visits focused particularly on that aspect to confirm the idea. Progressive focusing resulted in the research activity moving away from the general, i.e. descriptions of the environment to the specific that is looking more carefully at information exchange.

Typologies were also used to add order and logic to a mass of information and the guidance offered by Lofland (1971) was particularly helpful in this respect. An example of this technique is in the typology of handovers. Clarifying 'rules' was a similar technique and detailed analysis of the field notes led to the so-called 'Rules of Admission' to the labour ward which are explained in Chapter 5.

The data were analysed according to standard ethnographic techniques. The guidance offered by Lofland and Lofland (1984) and Hammersley and Atkinson (1983) were followed. All the data recorded in the fieldwork notes, the reflective diary, the analytic memos as well as transcripts of interviews and notes of other relevant documentation were copied and assembled. The data were inspected, read and reread, line by line until forty-three distinct themes emerged. The themes were coded and indexed. All the field notes were photocopied and with the use of a highlighter pen and scissors the notes were allocated to individually labelled envelope files. Each file had a theme title and a collection of copied, highlighted and edited field notes.

It became necessary at this point to arrange for further visits to each of the maternity units, in order to clarify and confirm omissions in the fieldwork notes. Sometimes the notes in the diary were unclear and they had to be correlated with the field notes for that day or night visit. Sometimes other documents, such as the ward message book, were used to confirm the field notes. It gradually became clear that there were overlapping and interconnecting themes and that a computer programme may be more efficient at analysis than my laborious long-hand method. The data in each file were then reconsidered and carefully reread line by line with minute attention to the detail of the text. The frustrations of poor handwriting or incomplete details were considerable but the problems could be overcome by cross-reference with another source, usually the diary.

The technique of progressive focusing was adopted. This is the specification, development and testing of problems/issues over the course of the fieldwork. This process continued after the fieldwork had formally ended.

Naturally a study of this nature had to be contained within a clearly defined time-scale and this necessarily limited the theory it generated.

It would be wrong to assume that each study only generates one theory but in this study there are aspects of many practice based theories. Descriptions are offered and meaning sought to explain the everyday activities of the midwife. This in itself is adding to the theoretical knowledge about midwives and the way they work. The analysis enabled the process by which they work, and their environment, to be carefully explored so as to inform, unravel and understand them and their social meaning.

Chapter 4

Some aspects of labour ward culture

■ The setting

This section describes in some detail the environment where the study took place. As previously explained the study was conducted in two maternity units. In order to preserve the anonymity of both units the descriptions presented and the incidences described are drawn from field notes written after visits to both hospitals. This 'fictitious' maternity unit, a combination of Hospital B and Hospital C, I have called the Valley Maternity Hospital.

The first day of fieldwork dawned and I telephoned the hospital to check that it was still convenient for me to attend. The switchboard operator rang the labour ward office. There was no reply, I asked her to keep trying as I was sure there would be someone there. 'They don't answer if they are busy' she said. I decided to visit anyway and considered what meaning I should attach to her comment. This aspect is explored more fully in Chapter 6, 'Aspects of Communication'. The Valley Hospital was part of a large district general hospital and was situated on the outskirts of a small town, serving the needs of a wide range of social classes in the area. There were also on the site a casualty department and paediatric unit, as well as the usual medical and surgical wards and theatres. There were a post-graduate medical centre and library, a school of nursing and midwifery and the usual facilities of libraries, visual aids, etc. There were a number of nurses' homes, medical staff residences and laboratory facilities.

The hospital was built on a sloping site, so once inside the building, the observer experienced differences in the levels, e.g. there was a door on the ground floor which opened on to a corridor which exited on the first floor of the main hospital. This seemed unreasonably confusing during the initial visits. It contributed to the feeling of disorientation commonly associated with being in a strange environment.

The Valley Maternity Hospital had approximately 4500 deliveries per year. There were twenty antenatal beds, twenty-four post-natal beds, ten delivery rooms and a special-care baby unit with fourteen special-care cots and four intensive-care cots. It also had an obstetric 'flying squad' which convened on demand and was available to attend any community obstetric emergency in the locality.

In the grounds of the hospital there was evidence of extensive building works. There were 'motorway cones' and fenced off 'holes' in the road. Opposite the entrance to the maternity unit there was evidence of large-scale building works, with scaffolding, piles of sand, cement mixers and two wheelbarrows. Those entering the maternity unit were directed around the side of the building, and had to negotiate a series of muddy puddles and broken paving stones.

When I arrived it was raining, there was an ambulance parked outside, and in the doorway, sheltering from the rain, were two ambulance men sharing a joke and a cigarette. They smiled and nodded towards me. I felt that I desperately needed a bundle of neatly photocopied questionnaires. I was unnerved by my blank notebook and vague ideas about continuity of care. I felt much more like a midwife than a researcher. I urgently needed to become familiar and at ease in this unit. The warnings from the literature to 'treat the familiar as strange' and play the role of 'a socially acceptable incompetent' rang in my ears. This was not going to be easy.

I walked along the corridor towards a central reception area. I was passed by a student nurse and a nursing auxiliary. They did not approach me. I wanted to turn back. I paused. I was trying to find the senior midwives' office and stopped to look for signs and notices to guide me. There were many notices (this is discussed later in this chapter) but none that would help me. I wondered what to do next. As I entered the unit it seemed an old building. I arrived and expected to find a clean, ordered, bustling maternity unit. However, it was dingy, untidy and in need of fresh paint and added to the paraphernalia of a busy maternity unit, there were the trappings of Christmas trees, tinsel, trimmings and holly. I was surprised to discover that it was built comparatively recently. It was in a very poor state of decorative repair, the walls were dirty and desperately needed painting. There was a nursery rhyme border which was badly faded and torn in many places. There was also an abundance of notices, mostly hand-written and secured to the walls with sellotape or dressing plaster. The corridor was carpeted but it seemed dirty. As I walked down the corridor I noticed a 'very pregnant' woman walking towards a door marked 'day room'. It was full, there were no seats left unoccupied and eight or so pregnant women sat surrounded by cigarette smoke. The television was on but no one seemed to be watching it. The day room was a dismal room with ancient magazines and well-worn chairs, the carpet was marked with cigarette burns and it was impossible to see out of the window. There was a video player linked to some promotional material but this was not in use. The walls had some posters but these had been disfigured with graffiti. There was a notice advertising the hospital radio and a very full notice board with private advertisements for used baby equipment and clothes. It seemed a sad room where the women went to smoke and wait. They waited either for labour or to go home.

On the ground floor were two dimly lit corridors, a noisy and ancient lift and a set of stone stairs which led to the first floor which was in a similar poor state of repair and seemed dirty. It was close to Christmas and as well as the general trappings of a busy maternity unit, the wards and corridors were beginning to be decorated with a variety of Christmas decorations. There were always rubbish bags, Central Sterile Supplies Department (CSSD) bags and linen bags piled in the corridor awaiting collection. At the time I began the fieldwork, the special-care baby unit was undergoing refurbishment, so pre-term and ill babies were being cared for in a ward close to the labour ward, which had been modified for that purpose.

There are frequent references in my field notes to aspects of the tidiness and cleanliness of the Unit. The overall impression was of a maternity unit that was in a poor state of repair. The unit always seemed very busy, there was always activity as all sorts of people walked purposefully in all directions.

I was lost, when a domestic assistant, in a familiar coloured uniform smiled and walked towards me. She wore rubber gloves and carried a bucket. She looked tired and worn, and smelled strongly of stale tobacco. 'Can I help, luv?' she said. Relieved, I said I was looking for Mrs P's office. She pointed down the corridor. 'Third door on the right, she doesn't bite.' I smiled and thought, 'have I located a "key informer" so soon?' There was no turning back. Some of the comments recorded in field notes (FN 4.1) enhance the description.

The corridors were frequently very full of various pieces of equipment. Alongside the intravenous infusion bottles were rubbish bags, pharmacy store boxes, dirty linen awaiting collection and empty cardboard boxes. There were empty cylinders of anaesthetic gas and full ones waiting to be fitted to the various types of apparatus. There was a row of hooks on the wall where the staff hung their outdoor coats, together with plastic aprons and gowns. Intermingled were various white coats which did not seem to belong to anyone in particular. On one visit, the corridor was almost totally blocked by a bed which had a notice, informing anyone who read it, that a wheel was broken. Alongside the admission-room door was a wheelchair, this was covered with a disposable, but soiled, waterproof pad. Outside the sluice room was a row of clean plastic aprons. There was a box of face masks on the shelf, but only once did I see these being used.

I walked down the dark corridor and knocked on the door. Mrs P. opened the door and greeted me warmly. It was clear she did not see me as the 'acceptable incompetent' but accepted that I was new, at least, to research. We talked about the difficulties in obtaining access and I reassured her as to the confidentiality of my findings and explained that I would use random initials to describe those whom I interviewed. I also confirmed that I would be sure to seek permission from the woman, her partner and the midwife before any observation.

Mrs P. said she would escort me on a tour of the Valley Maternity Unit. I put on my white coat and decided to avoid bringing a handbag in future. We walked along a dimly lit corridor towards the labour ward. At that moment Mrs P's bleeper went off and she rushed away to answer it.

FN 4.1

'The Unit is dirty again. The ashtray in the office is full of cigarette ends'.

'I arrived at the Unit at 12.30p.m. It looked untidy and disorganised as usual. The corridor was full of rubbish bags. There was a crate of empty intravenous infusion bottles and a sweeping brush.'

'I observed the usual state of untidiness and the obvious lack of storage space. As usual the corridor was littered with linen bags.'

'I nearly tripped over a rubbish bag on the way in today.'

'The labour ward bin bags were overflowing. Swabs and wrappings from the delivery packs were on the floor.'

'I am sitting on a stool in the corner of the delivery room, it has blood stains on the legs of the stool.'

'The trolley standing in the sluice, that had just been cleaned, 'very quickly' by the nursing auxiliary has blood stains on the wheels.'

'The unit is still dirty. The staff midwives sit and yawn. There is blood on the trolley, the stools and the sink unit.'

'The staff wore dirty plastic aprons. Although there was a good supply of these, they did not appear to change them when they were stained.'

'The admission room is full of equipment, there are boxes on the floors and in the corridor outside. There does not seem to be enough room for storage.'

'The labour ward office was its usual shambles. There were Christmas cards everywhere. On the table was a half-eaten cake with a sad satsuma and a tired tree bauble.'

■ Midwife or researcher?

I was alone, in a corridor, a midwife in a white coat with a notebook. Walking towards me was a woman. She was bent slightly forward with one hand holding her back and the other on her abdomen. She looked at me and said 'My husband has gone to park the bloody car. God knows where he is. What the hell shall I do now?' I knew at once that I had no option but to assist. It was clear she was in established labour and the gap between the contractions provided us both with the opportunity to try to find the labour ward. I was saved by my helpful domestic, Mrs M., who guided us both along the corridor, whispering words of encouragement to the woman as we went. I had arrived. My observation had begun and already I was wondering if the white coat was the best style of dress. Mrs P. reappeared, I was relieved, the labouring woman was delivered safely to the care of the midwives, and we resumed our tour of the unit.

The second floor was in a similarly poor state of repair. Here an auxiliary nurse, wearing green, was distributing disposable napkins, towels and gowns to a group of women. These women were all in night attire and standing around the trolley. I was introduced to the midwives and other staff. They looked a little confused, one asked if I would be filling in a questionnaire. Another wanted to know if I was anything to do with audit or the personnel department. I gave my standard explanation. There seemed to be a lot of people about. There were student nurses in yellow, student midwives in white, auxiliaries in green, midwives in white and Sisters in blue. The paediatricians were easy to recognise as they carried their stethoscopes around their necks like scarves. The obstetricians wore bow ties and the senior house officers looked untidy, unshaven and tired. The familiar on this occasion was not strange. I used my previous knowledge and experience to try to sort out what was happening.

The unit was very warm and had that distinctive smell associated with maternity units. The smell was difficult to describe but it was the warm smell of human beings combined with baby powder and clean laundry. It was recognisable as being a hospital maternity unit. The staff's humour and enthusiasm for their work struck me instantly, I felt at ease but not 'at home'. Later I visited the antenatal clinic and the special-care baby unit, but as the main focus of this study was the labour ward, descriptions of these areas are not included. The combined antenatal/post-natal wards were not included in the study although I visited these areas to conduct some interviews. The unit was a hive of activity. There was a feeling of energy and enthusiasm despite the poor physical environment. My tour took me next to the labour ward office.

■ The labour ward office

The labour ward office was the hub of life in the Valley Maternity Unit. It was the centre of all the activities. Unlike the rest of the delivery suite, this room was carpeted. Figure 4.1 illustrates its interesting shape. An office is usually a place dedicated to office work, i.e. writing, telephoning, arranging, managing, planning, filing and typing. This office witnessed some of those activities, but it was also a rest room, a snack bar, a common room, a waiting room and a treatment room. It was a real 'back-stage' area where many people came and went, and where the staff could, to quote a midwife, 'be themselves'.

Figure 4.1 The labour ward office

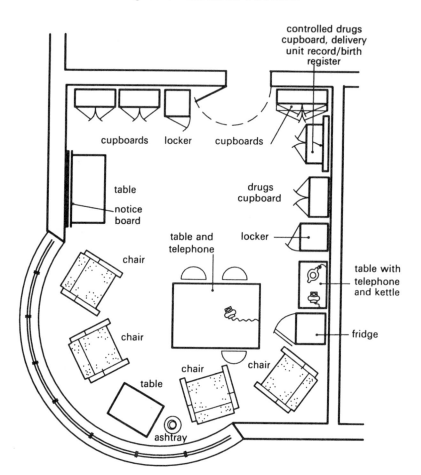

Women and their partners were positively discouraged from entering. If a woman arrived at the door, the staff would quickly jump up from their seats to deal with her before she had a chance to enter this 'hallowed' area.

Individuals of all grades wandered in and out without any apparent purpose. I observed doctors walk in and then just walk out. Sometimes they would stroll in, stare purposefully at the notice board, say nothing and walk out. Occasionally medical students would saunter in, look at me and before I had the opportunity to explain my purpose, amble out. The door was almost always open.

The staff sat in the office to write notes, to wait for work, to rest after a baby was born, to smoke, to talk, to answer the telephone, to eat and to drink. It was also the place where babies were given drugs and where controlled drugs were stored, counted and checked. It was the place where the staff handover took place. It was an informal classroom for student midwives. It was used for a variety of staff meetings, formal and informal. It was the place where the Sisters talked to the students to guide and counsel them and to fill in their report forms. It was the place where, behind closed doors, 'atrocity stories' as described by Dingwall (1977) were told and where the staff had 'post mortem' discussions (an informal review of the cases of the day).

It was the central reception area, the place where mothers presented themselves when they arrived in labour, and it was usually a bustling hive of activity. Radio 1 was usually playing in the background. Field note 4.2 introduces the more detailed description of the office.

FN 4.2

The main door of the office always seems to be open. In fact, today was the first time I had seen it closed. Two Sisters, one on day shift and one on night shift, closed the door to discuss a private matter. Just behind the door is a notice describing 'The Mechanisms of Labour'. This is the first time I have seen the notice. I leave the office, as the conversation is conducted in whispers. Afterwards one Sister said they enjoyed 'their chat' and often looked to each other for support especially when things went wrong. They both complained about the shortage of staff and openly discussed the faults of the manager.

At this time one Sister whom I had got to know very well said to me:

One good thing about this 'Know Your Midwife Scheme' is that the midwives are in working teams. You have to have a mate, you know – a friend to share what you are doing. It's awful on the community, sometimes there is no one to share your ideas with, it can be really lonely.

She had previously worked on the local 'Know your Midwife' pilot scheme, and also as a community midwife in the more conventional arrangements.

A place for sharing ideas and supporting each other was thus another function of the office.

During one visit I spent some time just looking carefully at the office and at what happened inside this room. In the office there were metal cabinets alongside the door (the doors of which were nearly always open). They contained bottles of squash, supplies of stationery, handbags, coats, books and equipment such as oxygen monitors. There did not seem to be any system but it was clear most of the midwives knew where to obtain particular items of equipment.

Next to the cupboards on the wall was a large, white board. Its function, which it served quite well, was to inform 'anyone' who came into the office:

(a) who was in labour and what stage of labour they were at.
(b) who was expected in.
(c) who was 'niggling' on the antenatal wards. (a term to be considered later).
(d) any 'high risk' cases who might need admission to the labour ward.

The board was full of in-house jargon, clearly understood by those who worked in the unit and illustrated examples of 'obstetric short hand'. It was clear that this was a very important piece of equipment.

Figure 4.2 shows how the board looked on the day of observation.

Technical terms are explained in the glossary but 'First Stage B' is one of the 'niggling rooms' to be considered later, and 'Messages: Anti D See Comm Book': refers to a notice in a book called the communication book where the attention of staff is drawn to a shortage of Anti D.

'Gravida 10, early labour', serves to warn the staff they may be called upon to conduct an emergency delivery.

Figure 4.2   The notice-board

ROOM	NAMES	
1	JL	In labour. Pethidine 100mg
2	AP	SROM. 37 week Pethidine 100mg Synto/F.S.E.
3	CP	Breech – Footling O Neg.
First Stage B	JW	Early Lab. Pethidine 100mg Short Stat. $N_2O + O_2$
Messages		Anti D – See Comm Book.
Gravida 10		Early Lab.
Mrs G. EDD – 25/12		– Expected
Mrs D. 34 Wks		– Expected

'Mrs G. EDD 25/12' means Mrs G whose baby is due on 25/12 is expected in.

'Mrs D 34 Wks' means the same except that Mrs D is 34 weeks pregnant and in pre-term labour. She would be likely to require greater precautions and preparations to be made. e.g. the room should be prepared with an extra heater and an incubator is switched to be warm at the time of the birth.

There were felt tip pens on the ledge under the board and an eraser. Any-one it seemed could write on the board, including the domestic, who would leave 'notes' about ordering rubber gloves and the state of the buckets.

■ Everyday rituals

After the mother was delivered and the case notes completed, the midwife, with some ceremony, would wipe that mother's name from the board. It appeared that this was the final act in completing the work. On one occasion two students appeared to quarrel over who would have the job of wiping the board clean of the name of a woman who had had a particularly difficult labour and birth. According to Roth (1978) a ritual is a formal action following a set pattern which expresses – through a symbol – a shared meaning. Cleaning the board is an example of a ritual; everyone working on the labour ward knew and understood that 'the case' had been dealt with. The baby had been delivered, the woman and her baby safely transferred to the post-natal ward, and the responsibility no longer rested with the midwives working on the labour ward. So the midwife, with relief and some drama, ceremoniously cleaned the board. The task was complete.

Drug-checking at the end of a shift was another ritual. The drugs stored in a white cupboard were counted and the numbers recorded. The midwife signed her name. This was the symbolic end of their period of responsibility. As Firth (1981) points out rituals are helpful in marking boundaries. Drug-counting is a ritual which marks the end of a shift. Whatever the pressure of work, the board was carefully kept up to date and served as a visual account of the unit's workload. A register of deliveries was also kept and was a permanent record of the number of 'cases' each shift had dealt with. This would be left open and on display at all times.

■ Statements and symbols

To return to the office, next to the board were four easy chairs, on and around which were more shopping bags and handbags. On the floor were lunch boxes, a pot of yoghurt and a women's magazine. On the table were a box of matches and some cigarettes.

All over the windows were Christmas cards; some were from the day staff to the night staff and vice versa. There were cards from doctors, the pharmacy, the pathology laboratories, as well as thirty-five cards from grateful patients and their families. The staff told me that 'Thank You' cards were generally viewed as a guide to the level of consumer satisfaction. The more letters and cards that were received the more sure were the staff that they were performing well. Many cards on display were quite old, referring to babies delivered more than four months previously. There was also a poem written by a grateful mother. On the window-sill were twelve potted plants, some of which seemed in a better state of health than others. There were two notices on the window-sill. One said:

'The Best Man for the Job is a Woman'

and the other:

'Smoking is My Business'.

I found these two notices particularly interesting. I wanted to know what was being said by those who place the notices. The first one I discovered was bought and placed in the office by a new midwife, whom the other midwives described as a 'bit of a feminist'. In my discussions with the midwives there were frequent mentions of their opinions that their job, and in particular, those aspects they described as the 'best bits' were taken over by the (usually) male doctors. Although a clearly articulated feminist perspective did not exist amongst this group of midwives, there was evidence of a move towards assertiveness and the reclaiming of their position. This notice, and some of the discussions, reflected these trends. Midwives were becoming less content with the system, especially when they felt they could do it better than the junior doctors, who were usually male. The second notice was, I discovered, purchased by a midwife who smoked. When I spoke to her about it, she told me that she was 'fed up' with people telling her that smoking was bad. She explained that she smoked because it helped her to cope with the pressures of her job, she was angry with those she called the 'healthy-living brigade' and explained that just because she was a midwife it did not mean she had to be a paragon of virtue.

On the table was a half-eaten chocolate cake, with the crumbs spilt off the plate onto the table. There was an empty plate with a knife which obviously previously contained toast, and a Christmas tree bauble. There was an almost-empty bottle of wine, with a label around the neck signed by the Consultant Obstetrician. There were a half eaten packet of biscuits and eight used cups or mugs and saucers. On the desk was a Kardex (nursing record file) and a set of notes. There were other notes in a wooden folder alongside the white board on the opposite wall. The desk also had a plastic folder with papers inside. There were a few pens, a punch and some paper clips. There was a plastic bag containing two specimen bottles which appeared to contain blood, together with a completed pathology laboratory form. The telephone was on the table and above it on the wall were detailed instructions as to how to summon medical and paediatric aid in an emergency. There were two more diagrams on the wall, one explained the dilatation of the cervix in a primigravida and the other dilatation of the cervix in a multigravida. These were provided by the School of Midwifery for student midwives. On the notice board were memos about off-duty arrangements and the opening and closing of departments during the Christmas holiday. There was also a hand-written notice asking for clean old tights or stockings, perhaps someone was making soft toys. The notice board also had details of the doctors' rota system and on-call arrangements.

Above the refrigerator was another large white board which listed the names of student midwives in training. There was alongside each name a grid, where ticks were added as each student completed a delivery or vaginal examination; a full row of ticks usually denoted a senior student midwife, who had completed the experience required for her training. Along the wall, on the other side of the desk, was the fridge. This contained a mixture of specimen bottles which were to be stored at a low temperature and various food items such as milk, butter and yoghurt. Above the fridge were a kettle, a jar of coffee, tea bags, milk, sugar and more cups.

Alongside the fridge was another wall-mounted cupboard, which was locked, but not labelled. The staff explained that someone had lost the key to the cupboard so it was never used. Next to this cupboard was a white wall-mounted cupboard which was used to store drugs. These drugs were controlled drugs and could be abused. They were carefully stored. This cupboard was locked and contained a second cupboard within the cupboard. The keys to this cupboard were held by the person in charge of the unit.

Below this cupboard was a sloping shelf which contained the birth register. This was a large book about 3'6" long and 2' high. It was opened out on this shelf and contained the details of the recent births within the unit. The births were usually recorded in chronological order unless someone entered a name too soon. When that happened the midwife in charge appeared to take control of the book and with some sticky labels obliterated the offending entry. It seemed very important that this book recorded births in the correct order.

Above the cupboard was a set of light switches and some red light bulbs which were seen to be flashing at regular intervals. As the light flashed, so the alarm bells sounded. This light did not produce an instant response, but the staff did move towards the delivery room eventually. The staff explained that the system was faulty and the lights would flash without anyone pressing a bell.

There was a folder above the switches, labelled:

Information on Planned Home Deliveries.
Please keep on labour in case of flying squad needs.

I noted this folder contained details instructing midwives on the procedure to be adopted if the 'flying squad' was called out but the label did not make clear to me the purpose of this document or how I should make use of its contents in an emergency. The midwives to whom I spoke were quite clear and unperturbed by the ambiguities apparent to an outsider.

The staff commented on how much they like the office and how it compared with offices in other maternity units. It was unusual in terms of its size: in other units the office may be small or the activities described conducted in various other places, e.g. staff sitting-rooms, kitchens, seminar/study rooms.

Valley Maternity Unit office was also unusual in that all the key activities associated with the unit were more likely to take place there. No one, it seems, was really responsible for the office. On one occasion I observed it being cleaned by a domestic assistant and once it was rearranged and 'tidied' by the Sister-in-charge. All staff appeared to have equal right of entry. As previously mentioned, women as 'patients' were discouraged from entering.

To summarise, the office was the centre of the labour ward activity, it was busy, yet a haven of tranquillity after the emotion and stress of the delivery room. It was the meeting-point and the safe area in a traumatic working environment. It had many and varied functions, it was used for administrative purposes, the paper work, as a sitting room, a restaurant, a picnic area, a drug storage area, a clinical treatment room, a classroom, a board room, a committee room, a consulting and counselling room, a reception room, a storage room, a locker room, kitchen and staff room.

It was a private area away from the public gaze and yet it remained within the public sphere of the hospital. It was an area where the staff could relax, be themselves, comment on the management of cases, confess to their inadequacies and to the mistakes that might have been made. It was a therapeutic, back-stage area which did not conform to the public rules of hygiene and order which characterised the public space of a hospital.

Curtis (1992) writing on clinical supervision in midwifery practice says:

Intergroup communication underpins the development of cultural norms and is an essential element of the assimilation of new practitioners as they enter specific work settings.

She describes how individuals entering from other practice areas learn what is preferred, what is tolerated and what is frowned upon. The labour ward office at Valley Maternity Unit was that area where cultural norms were established, where intergroup communication was well-practised. Supervision as an activity that supported the sometimes-isolated practitioner (even in the labour ward) was carried out. It was clearly an area where the midwives were comfortable, were nurtured physically and emotionally and enabled to continue to carry out their demanding task. It was also the site of the production of a collective identity.

■ The delivery room: the inner sanctum

I called the delivery room 'the inner sanctum' because it seemed that, at first, the midwives were reluctant to let me in. Despite their knowledge of my background and the fact that I had obtained 'official approval' they tended to view me as an intruder. On another occasion I was approached by a midwife, who had missed my explanation, and asked if I was 'medical'. She said, 'Look, we can't just let anyone in here – it's like a "fair" already'. They were initially happy to let me look carefully at an unoccupied room but were hesitant at granting total access.

The delivery room itself was viewed much more as a special and intimate area where the midwife and the woman went to some lengths to withdraw and protect themselves from the public. The delivery room had a special feel and I understood the midwives' reluctance to include this area in the 'free for all' public areas.

Interestingly, the delivery rooms were usually much cleaner and better organised than the office and corridor areas. The rooms were quite small and tightly packed with equipment. The outer door had a notice which advised those entering to 'knock and wait'. This was usually ignored by midwives and doctors working on the unit, but 'outsiders' such as myself and the medical students usually obeyed.

Two of the rooms were considerably warmer than the others: these rooms were reserved as far as possible, for use when pre-term or other small babies were expected. Figure 4.3 shows how much equipment was packed into a very small room. Field note 4.3 gives the comments I made at the time.

FN 4.3

The delivery rooms are quite bright and cheerful. The windows have curtains with clouds and rainbow patterns and the walls generally look in a better state of repair. These rooms are excessively hot especially if the researcher is inappropriately dressed.

I spoke to the midwives and students about the delivery rooms and their comments are recorded in Field note 4.4.

Figure 4.3 The delivery room

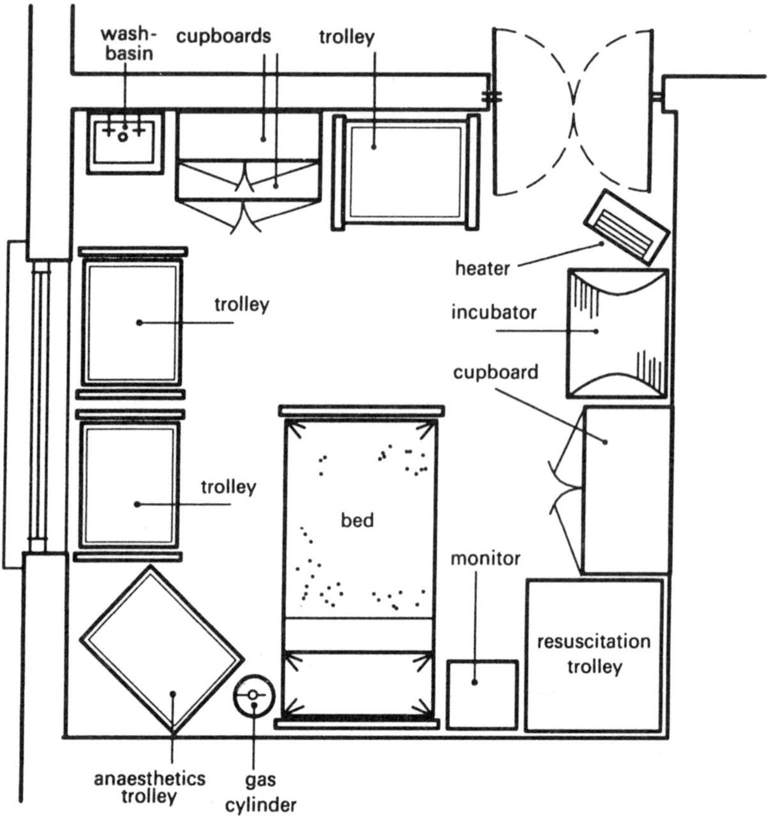

FN 4.4

Yes, the rooms are quite nice really.

There is not enough room, you see – if anyone wants to squat or anything its hopeless.

You get used to the heat, its not so bad really.

It would be nice to get some better equipment you know, bean bags.

I find the rooms are terribly small. They are so clinical, just like an operating theatre, the curtains are a gesture to the natural childbirth movement. It is difficult to do any sort of delivery except the conventional dorsal or lithotomy position. It's a joke really, they are really too small.

Squatting is an alternative position for delivery (see Balaskas, 1983). Women who chose, or were advised by the midwife, to try a more upright position for labour and/or the birth often found that the tightly packed delivery room was much too small. There was insufficient space to put a mattress on the floor or to facilitate the use of a bean bag. Many women were very uncomfortable lying on the hard delivery room bed, especially if they were connected by wide elastic straps to a fetal monitoring machine and would have preferred to lie on a bean bag, or kneel on a mattress on the floor.

The comment 'a gesture to the Natural Childbirth Movement' is interesting as it reflects the struggle for the control of care during birth and indeed the place of birth. The midwives seemed aware of the historical conflict between the medical profession and midwives (Donnison, 1977; Oakley, 1984). The midwives to whom I spoke commented that they viewed the introduction of curtains and soft furnishings as a cosmetic exercise. They told me that they saw this as an attempt to placate those who were striving for more natural childbirth. They felt that the efforts being made to 'humanise the labour ward' and make it more home-like were merely gestures to organised and vocal consumer demands. Some agreed that it made for a more pleasant working environment but some dismissed it as tokenism.

One comment made by a midwife reflects well how some midwives viewed their work: it is recorded in Field note 4.5.

FN 4.5

You see they have got it all wrong. They spend money on curtains and bean bags . . . but we don't get any more staff.

I'm in favour of home births – it must be better than running around here – going from one to another – just catching the babies.

I think they think they can buy off women with a few curtains and some Laura Ashley wallpaper, what they don't realise is that more and more women are waking up and realising that they want is good care, with the same midwife anywhere.

The delivery room was a special place and only with some reluctance did the midwives allow anyone other than the woman and her partner to enter these rooms. The window on the door was blocked and callers were discouraged. It could not be like the bedroom in a home birth but many midwives felt that they should be striving towards achieving something similar.

Access to the inner sanctum had to be earned and it was not until I had spent some two weeks or so on observational visits that the atmosphere relaxed enough to discuss my being present during labour and birth. I had decided to ask if I could wear theatre dress. These pale blue and green trouser suits were readily available and often worn by the midwives, particularly those who were involved in caring for women during prolonged labour. The Sister in charge readily agreed and appeared relieved to see me discard the white coat. I had to forego the note pad but by this stage I was getting better at writing one or two words as prompts in a much smaller notebook. The dictaphone slotted easily into the pocket in the theatre top and could be used in off-stage areas (e.g. the toilet and the changing rooms) to record details. The change of clothes certainly appeared to help in obtaining access to the inner sanctum, as did the staff's increasing understanding of me and the nature of my research. Access is never guaranteed in fieldwork settings, it has to be negotiated and earned.

The delivery rooms were unique and completely different from the more public areas of the office, corridors and the wards.

■ Notices

The Valley Maternity Hospital had a plethora of notices. As a stranger to the unit, trying to make sense of a new environment I read and reread the notices, like a traveller in a strange city, looking carefully for guidance and clues to the environment. As an ethnographer looking at the culture of a hospital maternity unit I could not ignore these notices. What could they tell me about Valley Maternity Hospital, how could the notices help me to seek meanings in this social world?

Most hospitals have lots of notices which are there to inform or to guide strangers to the building and its departments. There are usually notices telling people where to wait or where to leave specimens. Valley Maternity Hospital was distinctive in the vast quantity of notices and in the seemingly haphazard way they were fixed to the walls. Most were untidily hand-written and fastened to walls with large quantities of sellotape or the more expensive variety of sticking plaster. The notices formed part of the variety of documentary materials that was available for the researcher. Some notices were formal, printed and carried the authority associated with either the health authority or professional organisation or trades union. There were various notices issued by the School of Midwifery which gave information about student midwives. Additionally there were very many informal notices which contributed to the environment at Valley Maternity Hospital.

It was felt that the notices were useful as a source of 'sensitising concepts' (Blumer, 1954). They suggested ways in which the staff on the labour ward organised the work, maintained control of the environment and asserted their authority. The notices also served to set the agenda for discussion and prompted further investigation of the subject of the notice.

There was a notice about the management of ruptured membranes. This prompted much interesting discussion. There were many examples of notices which illustrated where an individual had an axe to grind, e.g. the notices in the sluice and the paediatric on-call system.

The notices were particularly interesting in that they furnished the researcher with information about the setting which would otherwise be difficult to obtain. They represented public statements on the beliefs and values of the organisation. They were a picture of the world of Valley Maternity Hospital.

The notices were frequently the starting-point for discussion on other aspects of life in the labour ward, e.g. 'no more off duty requests for next week' and 'All patients must be seen by the SHO before discharge'. In order to present the information contained on the notices it was necessary to construct a typology of notices.

Notices can be divided into three distinct categories:

(a) negative or 'do not' notices;
(b) request notices;
(c) informative or instructive notices.

□ **Negative notices**

These formed the largest section, and included:

1. Do *not* take drinks downstairs.
2. Patients and relatives from other ward are *not* allowed to use this machine.
3. Drinks are *not* to be carried into the wards.
4. Do *not* smoke.
5. *No* admission to unauthorised persons.
6. Do *not* use the phone at night. Patients sleeping.
7. Do *not* enter.
8. Do *not* ring the bell unless you want to come in.
9. Do *not* stub out cigarettes on the floor.

□ **Request notices**

1. Please do not put cups on the floor. Place in bins provided. (This notice has a negative flavour but is prefaced with please.)
2. Please empty buckets after use as standing water encourages germs – signed, Sally.

   Sally is a nursing auxiliary. This notice is in the sluice, obviously her domain. She explained that 'smelly buckets' were the bane of her life, particularly when the labour ward had been busy. It is also worthy of comment that Sally, the auxiliary does not require the signature of the midwife to add credence to her request. Does this reflect the division of labour in the labour ward? It is also interesting that the lay term 'germs' is acceptable in the sluice area.

3. If the baby is ill, leave a long bit of cord for Dr A.
   (This notice has no other explanation.)
4. Smoking is my business.
   (On labour ward office desk.) This notice is discussed in the previous section.
5. Please knock and wait.
   (Usually ignored.)
6. Please do not ask for change for coffee machine.
7. Please wash up your cups after use.
8. Please ask the paper man to call on the labour ward when he arrives.
9. Don't forget labour ward when the bun trolley comes.
10. Off-duty requests by today or forget it.

□ **Informative notices**

1. Pudendal needles are not disposable.
2. Visiting times are from . . .
3. Only two visitors per bed.
4. The mechanism of labour.
   (This is a large chart designed for students.)
5. Dilatation of the Cervix,
   Primigravida
   Multigravida.
   (This notice is behind the office door, therefore rarely seen.)
6. Information on Planned Home Deliveries.
7. For Flying Squad calls please note that there are three drug boxes to be collected.
8. The principles of Fetal Monitoring.
   (This is a large chart, published by the manufacturer of monitoring equipment designed to demonstrate abnormalities of fetal heart trace.)
9. No more off-duty requests for next week.
10. All 'patients' to be seen by SHO before discharge.

As the study progressed I observed that there had been a new series of notices in the unit. I discussed them with Sister B. who was in charge. She told me that because of the turnover of staff there were more people working in the unit who did not know the 'routines'. She explained that more notices were required to ensure that everybody knew what the consultants wanted and how to respond in an emergency. There was very rarely any public debate about what the consultants wanted, the notice appeared to indicate compliance.

The new notices included:

1. If you need a paediatrician from 9–5 pm, Monday–Friday, please ask for SCBU paeds.
   At other times it is the 'on call' paeds.
2. All patients to have immediate ECTG run on admission even if they are only in for one hour.
3. Please photostat cooperation cards of mothers who have prem. babies, very ill babies, SBs or NND.
   Prem = born too early.
   SBs = still-born infants.
   NND = Neonatal Death
4. All patients with SROM, regardless of gestation if not in active labour, are not to have VEs unless contraindicated. Speculum only.

Some notices were clearly aimed at the professional and auxiliary staff employed in the unit, whilst other notices seemed reserved for what I called in my field notes 'The enemy'. It appeared that the notices to the public did not usually offer courtesy and respect but were rather authoritarian in tone. It might be suggested that the notices were to signify aspects of control or to make clear who was in charge. When I read the public notes, as an outsider, I felt intimidated and most anxious not to cause offence or break any rules.

■ A utonomy and the midwife

I spoke to the midwives on the unit about 'the notices' and in particular those most recently included. I spoke to the permanent Sister-in-charge on the labour ward. This interview was particularly informative. She told me that she had always viewed herself as an independent practitioner in cases of normal childbirth. She had worked for many years as a community midwife. She moved into the hospital for many reasons but chiefly because 'normal birth had moved back into hospital'. She felt that at Valley Maternity Hospital all pregnancies fell under medical management and were, as Percival (1970) said, 'normal only in retrospect'. She felt that she was now no longer a practitioner in her own right but an obstetric nurse and 'medical man's handmaiden' or 'minder of machines'. She went on to explain that she and the midwives who worked on the unit were attempting to reclaim some of the responsibility. She explained how the notice detailing action to be taken on spontaneous rupture of membranes now includes the phrase 'unless contraindicated'. She said that she insisted the phrase was included, so that midwives made the decisions: 'We use the notices to show we are in control. We are in a battle which we will win, but not yet.' The battle referred to was the battle against the medicalisation and the hospitalisation of childbirth. The other ongoing battle is the one in which midwives are fighting to regain their professional autonomy which some argue was lost when the place of birth became the hospital. Thus the midwives aim to present themselves as competent practitioners. They use appropriate language, e.g. 'unless contraindicated', to convey their abilities and their experience and to control their situation. Notices are more than providers of information. They are also there to set parameters of authority.

The notices served to guide me to other areas of interest, and in particular to the way that the midwives endeavoured to exert some form of control over their environment. The Sister also explained how notices often appeared in response to an 'untoward incident' (see Field note 4.6).

FN 4.6

Take that notice about all patients to be seen by an SHO before discharge.

It's rubbish. That is there because one day last week a patient came in and was not doing much. She hung around for a bit and nothing happened. The pains went, she had no show. Membranes intact. She had a run (a period of fetal heart monitoring) and the fetal heart was fine. She wanted to go home, she had a 2-year-old who was staying with her mother-in-law and she couldn't stand her mother-in-law. One of the midwives examined her. She was a multips os.* We let her go home. Guess what! That's right she delivered in the ambulance on the way back in. Everything was okay, mother and baby were fine. But what happens? The standard knee-jerk response. It must be our fault. So a junior SHO, still wet behind the ears, has to give his okay for her to go. That makes it alright, they think. I'll take the notice down next week and we will go back to normal.

---

* In the primigravida the external os remains closed until labour is well advanced and the cervix is flattened against the presenting part and completely effaced. In the multigravida (often referred to colloquially as multips) the external os begins to dilate before effacement is complete. This often occurs before labour is well established. Hence multips os: the definition of the cervix of a woman who has previously had a child and is not yet in labour in this pregnancy.

Descriptions of the environment and the culture are a very important part of any ethnographic study. This chapter has presented a picture of life in a British maternity hospital in the late 1980s. It forms the backdrop for the chapters that follow.

Chapter 5

All in a day's work

■ Admissions

Parsons (1951) described four main behaviour patterns to which a person must conform in order to be socially defined as sick. He argued that the sick person is obliged to accept that he (or she):

1. is relieved of his/her normal duties;
2. is not responsible for his/her condition and is unable to cure himself/herself;
3. is in an undesirable condition and must get well;
4. is expected to seek medical help.

I would argue that throughout the period of my research, alongside the hospitalisation, medicalisation and increasing intervention in birth, women were led into the role of sick person. The system required a woman to attend the hospital and although she was often capable of continuing with light domestic duties attendance for admission relieved her of this opportunity. Women admitted in labour would be referred to as 'patients' and symbolically the responsibility for themselves and their condition was packed into a large plastic bag labelled 'Patients' Property'. With the hospital white gown, offered to save soiling the woman's own nightdress, the woman would abdicate responsibility for herself. It could be argued that labour is an undesirable condition, to be got through, in order to get well again. A desire to accelerate normal labour by the use of artificial rupture of the membranes and the use of intravenous syntocinon to stimulate uterine action would support the theory of the undesirable condition, with the cure being birth. Even syntometrine was said to be used in the third stage of labour 'to shorten the third stage' as if there was some urgency to end this undesirable condition. As Chapters 1 and 2 have indicated, women are of course expected to seek medical help in this 'abnormal condition.'

This section describes the events that occurred around the time of admission. It demonstrates how women adopted the role of the patient and how the midwives took this opportunity to take control of the situation.

The admission procedure was a very important activity. It was at this stage that the midwife decided the subsequent management and care of the woman. If she made an incorrect decision this could interfere with the organisation and control of the work. This aspect is explained in more detail in Chapter 6 'Getting through the work'.

The women who arrived at the delivery suite were, in most cases, expected. During the antenatal period the women would be encouraged to telephone the labour ward prior to admission so that the antenatal notes could be obtained and the staff warned of their impending arrival. Leaflets available to women always included a list of 'When to ring the hospital!'

Some women did not ring. This may be because they forgot, or did not have access to a telephone. Some women would telephone to arrange for an ambulance to bring them in, but this practice was generally discouraged, unless the midwife felt it was an emergency. An obstetric 'Flying Squad', which was convened on demand, could be sent out to any obstetric emergency that warranted intervention before admission. The obstetric flying squad consisted of an obstetrician, anaesthetist, paediatrician, a senior midwife and perhaps a student. They carried emergency equipment.

However, in the normal type of admission, the woman would be expected and the midwife and/or a student would meet her and her family at the main door to the delivery suite. The midwife usually looked at the woman and made an initial assessment of her condition. At this stage it was only a visual assessment.

In a survey of a large volunteer sample of women (Boyd and Sellars, 1982) several women mentioned their feelings of apprehension and anxiety on admission to the labour ward. This was supported by observation. It was clear that most women were anxious and often in pain. The women were usually greeted quite warmly. The staff usually said, 'Hello, Mrs ? How are you?'

The woman was then directed into the admission room. This room was quite large but was also used as a storeroom for sterile packs and other equipment. It was not a pleasant room and did little to create a relaxed atmosphere. The woman would be directed to undress and transfer the contents of her suitcase (if she had one) to a large white plastic bag. It was clear that in most cases the packing of the suitcase had been undertaken with some care. The night-clothes, slippers and toilet-bag would be neatly positioned in the case. Sometimes there would be some baby clothes, neatly ironed and packed in tissue paper. The toilet bag was often new with contents gleaming and untouched. Towels were neatly folded and the obligatory two large packets of sanitary towels would be positioned in the case.

The contents of the case, presumably lovingly and carefully packed at home would be deposited into a plastic bag. The woman would be advised that the case was now to contain her outside clothes. Like a prisoner stripped of her identity the woman, clad in an inadequate gown with a back opening, would be encouraged to bathe. As a convict is issued with a number, an identity bracelet also with a number would be attached to the woman's wrist. The depersonalisation procedure completed, the partner was instructed to take home the case and the contents and the woman's outside clothes, as soon as possible. He would be warned of the dangers of losing personal property and with a close of the lid the last means of escape disappeared. The woman had become a patient and part of the system.

Once the above procedure was completed the woman would be encouraged to lie on the couch in the admission room. The couch was high and narrow. It was very difficult for women to position themselves on the couch particularly during the latter stages of pregnancy. The woman, often left pink and breathless by the experience, would lie on the couch. The pains that had brought her in had often now subsided. Often I would hear the woman express her shame to her partner. 'All this trouble I've caused and now the pains have gone away!' The physiological explanation for the cessation of labour was not known but, like cows and mice, women when moved in labour often stop labouring. The nesting instinct it seems, requires peace, quiet and a feeling of safety. This was difficult to achieve in a formal hospital setting.

The midwife would then reappear and the conversation would often followed the pattern shown in Field note 5.1.

FN 5.1

Hello. Mrs Jones is it? (She confirms the name)

First baby?

What has been happening?

How often are the pains coming?

Have the waters gone?

Have you had a show?

Just pop along here.

Pop up on to the bed.

That's fine.

Baby moving all right today.

I'll just listen to the heart beat.

I'll just check your blood pressure.

Pop this thermometer into your mouth.

That's fine.

Hubby coming in?

The woman would reluctantly 'confess' to not having had any pains recently. The admission procedure usually involved a vaginal examination comparable with the vaginal examinations that form part of gynaecological examinations.

Richman and Goldthorpe (1977) in 'When was your last period?' present an account of some of the cultural features of the diagnostic processes in the setting of a gynaecological outpatients' clinic. Although their paper is concerned with the everyday aspects of making a gynaecological diagnosis, the references to vaginal examinations show an interesting similarity with midwifery practice:

> After offering an account of her troubles, the proceedings are suspended for the vaginal examination. Gynaecologists introduce this topic with talk represented by verbal formulae emphasising it as a mechanical event (Richman and Goldthorpe, 1977, p. 164).

This intrusive, even invasive procedure is handled by midwives as a mechanical and routine event. The admission procedure would follow a standard pattern, enemas and shaves were no longer used but a period of external monitoring was normal practice, after the production, of course, of the obligatory specimen of urine.

Other writers have commented that midwives and women in admission may have a different set of priorities at this time. Garforth and Garcia (1987) comment that the women may be concerned with the minutiae of admission, e.g. how the child at home is getting on with the neighbour; how much will it hurt; how will she cope; whilst the midwife's main concern is to discover what is happening and reassure herself that mother and baby were well. They go on to say that providing appropriate care for individual women with varying needs is a daunting task. This is particularly so when admission is often the first time the midwife and the woman concerned have met. Midwives have to establish a relationship with women very quickly.

It was normal practice to conduct a vaginal examination shortly after admission. The partner would be encouraged to leave and the midwife would say, 'Right, I'm just going to examine you inside Mrs J.' She would open a sterile pack and wash her hands. She would put on some sterile gloves then say 'Okay, ready now, bring your knees up, heels together and let your legs flop apart.' The woman would follow the instruction and stare at the ceiling. The midwife would sometimes chat about the weather as she prepared her equipment. The next sentence would always be 'I'm just going to wash you down.' Then the midwife would place green sheets and towels under the woman's buttocks and over her abdomen with a final towel draped around her leg. The midwife had created an artificial sterile field. Almost invariably the woman would now position her feet on top of the sheet. The midwife, often exasperated, would reprimand the woman for acting inappropriately. The woman, admonished, now knew who was in charge. The procedure continued. The midwife would slip her fingers into the vagina and say 'Just relax.'

Emerson (1970) describes how reality is sustained during gynaecological examinations. She describes, for instance, 'rituals of respects' and how they are used to express dignity for the patient. The patient's body is draped so as to expose only that part which is to receive the technical attention of the doctor (or in this case, the midwife). She records the doctor's soothing tone of voice: 'Now relax as much as you can, I'll be as gentle as I can.'

The procedure completed, the midwife would announce 'You are 2 centimetres (4 centimetres)' etc. Sometimes this was not followed by an explanation. Sometimes it was issued almost as a reprimand or with a sense of despair, 'You are only 3 centimetres' The plan of action was then decided. It was rare for the woman to be involved in the discussion at this stage.

Many women were clearly pleased to have the responsibility for their care taken out of their hands. After all, this was why they had come to hospital and this was what the experts who know best had decided. This phenomenon of 'they know what they're doing' was explored by Drayton and Rees (1984). The women in their study accepted routine if the obstetric and midwifery staff recommended it.

Firth (1981) writing in 'Medical Encounters', described some of the routines she encountered in a tropical diseases hospital. She comments on the strains of being 'a captive' within the hospital setting. Women and their partners often internalised the captive role and asked permission to leave the labour ward.

Women who arrived at the labour ward were anxious, distressed, frequently observed to be in pain and generally unsure about what was likely to happen to them. They were subjected to a routine procedure which began with the removal of their clothes and ended with them being rendered powerless and attached to a fetal heart-rate monitor.

Whilst there are often good midwifery and obstetric reasons for conducting a vaginal examination and making an accurate assessment of the woman's condition, one must speculate as to the rationale behind the practice of putting a woman to bed and rendering her a powerless captive of the hospital system. It was clear that the woman's and the midwives' priorities were very different at this time. The midwife viewed the woman – and dealt with her – as 'work'. It may be good 'work' or merely a time-consuming interruption. The admission procedure defined the work and began the process of socialising the woman into her new role as a hospital 'patient'. Other aspects of admission are explored on pages 96–9 and 102–4.

■ Birth: the labour process

Labour can be divided into three stages. The first stage is characterised by regular painful contractions and the opening-up of the cervix. The second stage begins when the baby is ready to be born and the cervix is fully dilated. This section describes the events that occurred at the time of birth.

It became clear that the second stage of labour and the delivery were viewed as the most important aspect of the midwives' work. When a woman was in the second stage of labour and was close to delivery the atmosphere on the labour ward changed considerably. There was an increase in tension, and something close to panic was expressed by the new student midwives. Across the corridor, a midwife would shout 'Can I have some help please? Mrs Smith is fully.' This was a commonly used abbreviation. The staff busied themselves, collecting trolleys, delivery packs, cots, injection trays, and those without one donned a clean plastic apron.

On some occasions, a midwife would rush into the office to make an urgent telephone call. Sometimes she would be ringing a missing partner, urging him to come straight away; sometimes she would be ringing for a doctor or asking for a paediatrician to be present for the delivery.

At this time tea would be left to go cold in the office and incoming admissions would be directed to the admission room by a nursing auxiliary. On more than one occasion, two or three women reached the second stage of labour at the same time. The atmosphere was quite electrifying. It was important at these times to keep out of everyone's way and yet still clearly observe the events.

The midwives strongly disliked these circumstances and frequently made comments such as these shown in Field note 5.2.

FN 5.2 —————————————————————————

'Its like a fairground.'

'. . . as usual, all or nothing.' 'feast or famine'

'What's the matter with these women today?'

'Why do they all "come off" at once?'

'Come off' was a new term to me, it meant, 'Why do they all deliver at the same time?'. The midwives explained to me that the tension around the time of birth was considerable. The job became instantly more demanding, some midwives became intolerant of student midwives and frequently appeared to resent the presence of the medical students. They strongly disliked medical intervention especially when the birth appeared to be going well. On one occasion I heard a midwife say to a junior house officer 'No, thanks, you are not wanted here, we will call you if and when we need you. Please go away.' As she closed the door she sighed and said 'Why do they always turn up when the hard work is done? You'll not catch them around for the dreary bits, only the drama.'

At the time of the delivery of the baby I usually chose to stay in one of the delivery rooms. It would have been even more disruptive to the women in labour to have a researcher join the stream of people who entered and left the room during the birth of the baby. On one occasion I counted a total of twenty people make a total of twenty-six entries and exits during one forty-minute period. This included the woman's partner, mother, sister, aunt and elder daughter, the house officer, the registrar, the paediatrician and the paediatric registrar, the anaesthetist, the operating department assistant, four midwifery sisters, two student midwives, a nursing auxiliary, a midwifery manager, and a researcher (me)!

I often spoke to the women after the birth of their baby. I was particularly interested in their perceptions of continuity and their feelings about birth. The women seemed to have very low expectations, as indicated by this comment by one woman who said to me about her experience of birth, 'I am still here and I have got a son. How can I ask for anything more?'

Another woman explained to me that although she had agreed that the student midwives could be present for the birth she was unnerved by what she described as 'the row of frightened faces in the small delivery room'.

Another woman said that she really liked it when the students were there because the midwife would tell them what was going on and she could listen too. The women in the Valley Maternity Hospital were indeed compliant.

■ Terms of endearment

I usually sat near the head of the bed and often assisted the midwife by passing equipment. As I sat and observed, I noted that there was a recognisable and frequently repeated list of well-meaning names and phrases used during each birth. Some of these terms of endearment are listed in Field note 5.3. In Eric Berne (1968) transactional analysis terms, the midwives frequently viewed the relationship with women in terms of parent/child which is also reminiscent of the Garmonikow classification of the social relations formed by the hospital. This further supported the theory that the midwives strove to achieve a degree of power and dominance over women yet the terminology was used in a warm and affectionate manner. The midwives were kind but frequently reminded me of parental figures.

FN 5.3

Come on, Sweetie Pie.	Carry on, lovey.
Well done, girlie.	Okay, *cariad**
Good girl.	There's nothing wrong with that
Love.	Joe Soap!**
Darling.	Pop along, lovely girl.
Poppett.	Really great, love.
Poppy.	Super girl.
That's fine, lovely.	Come on, lovely.
Well done, sweetheart.	Dear.
Babes.	Deary.
Baby.	My lovely Honeybunch.
My little one.	Scrunchbunch.
Lovely, Darling.	

---

* Cariad: a Welsh form of endearment; roughly translated it means 'love', or 'darling'.
** 'There is nothing wrong with that Joe Soap.' This phrase was uttered after the Sister had listened to the fetal heart beat. There had been some concern expressed about the rate of the heart beat, the Sister finished listening and patted the woman on the abdomen then she said: 'There is nothing wrong with that Joe Soap' – she was referring to the fetus and the fetal heart-rate.

I usually interviewed the women who had been in labour a day or so after the birth. I would chat about their experience and encourage them to 'tell it as it was'. Many women mentioned the pet names they had been called in labour. Two women said that they found the terminology both offensive and patronising. However most women seemed to accept that it was normal practice. One concluded: 'All midwives say things like that, don't they?'

The women also spoke about the difficulty in establishing a relationship with a midwife especially if she had only just arrived on duty. One woman said: 'I felt really sorry for the midwife. She didn't know me from Adam. I was 'high' on the gas. I couldn't help.' It was interesting to note how this woman appeared to feel responsible to the midwife for her 'failure'.

As previously explained the field notes were compiled soon after the visit. The following field note is reproduced in its entirety. It records the events that surrounded one woman's experience of birth and the comments I made in the field notes at the time. It was not untypical of the birth in that unit.

Field note 5.4 consists of notes taken during and shortly after the birth of the baby.

■ Emotional labour

Pam Smith (1992) describes the term 'Emotional Labour' as 'the unrecognised and unrewarded components of service sector work undertaken mainly by women.' The term was first used by Professor Arlie Hochschild, an American sociologist.

FN 5.4

Mrs C is well advanced in labour, as she exhales she makes a grunting noise which the midwives clearly recognise as a sign that the second stage of labour is approaching. They respond to this sign by encouraging her to lie on her side. The midwife peers at the anus. The woman's partner looks away. The midwife explains to the student that she is looking for signs that the cervix is fully dilated. She points out how the vulva is distended and together they peer anxiously waiting for a glimpse of the baby's head. With a triumphant shout of 'There it is', the Sister encourages the student to 'scrub up'. In practice this means a rather hurried hand wash with a surgical lotion. Sister turns to me and demonstrates that she views me as a fellow midwife by saying 'The medical students always make a meal of it, [scrubbing up] and come close to missing the case'. I laugh and enjoy being one of the cast. The student midwife washes her hands, the sterile packs are opened and she dons the rubber gloves. At the same time Sister, who is supervising the delivery, busied herself with the various tasks, whilst saying to the woman: 'Don't push yet love . . . we are not quite ready.'

The heater in the cot is switched on, the cord clamp and mucous extractor (to clear the baby's airways) are opened ready. On a small cardboard tray she collects a syringe, needle and an ampoule of the drug syntometrine (this is given to reduce the risk of bleeding during the third stage). The student is now ready, having prepared her trolley. She says to the woman: 'I'm just going to wash you down.'

They always use exactly the same words, a fuller explanation is never offered. She dips the swabs into warm disinfectant solution and washes the vulval area. This procedure is carried out with accurate precision. Five swabs are used and the area is washed from top to bottom and always in the same order. The abdomen and the area between and beneath the mother's legs is draped with clean sterile towels. The woman usually (somewhat distracted at this point), again lifts her feet and places them, incorrectly on the sterile towel. The woman is corrected and told that the area is kept clean ready for the baby. Now the student begins to give the woman instructions: 'Now, when the pain comes, take a deep breath in, hold your breath and push. Push right down into your bottom.' The woman nods her compliance, grips her partner's arm and begins to push. Sometimes she pushes harder than at other times. If her pushes are thought to lack effort the same comment is always made: 'Now, don't waste your pains, long hard pushes are better than short little ones.'

As time progresses the head advances, the woman is now given another instruction: 'Now then, in a little while I'm going to tell you not to push, but to pant. You know, in and out like a dog.' She does not tell the woman why this is necessary. Sometimes the woman nods and thus acknowledges the request. On other occasions she just rests back on the pillows, waiting for the next pain. 'Come along – another push: your face isn't red enough yet.' The woman looks confused again. The student asks the midwife: 'Does she need an episiotomy?' The woman looks up and looks alarmed. 'What's that?' Sister replies 'Oh, it's only a little cut, to help baby out – I think you will be all right.'

Another pain overtakes the woman and she pushes. The head crowns. 'Don't push, pant', screams the student as she attempts to control the delivery of the head. The woman does not acknowledge that she has either heard or understood the command.

'That's the head out' says the student.
'Feel for the cord', says the midwife.
The student checks that the umbilical cord is not trapped around the baby's neck. They wait. It is quiet. No one says anything.
'Do you want to see the baby's head' says the midwife.
The woman sits up 'Oh my God', she flops back down on the pillow 'There is another pain coming'.
She looks imploringly at the Sister, then at the student, then at me.
'Give another push then', says Sister.
She pushes, the head rotates, the shoulders appear. The baby is born. Sister gives an injection of syntometrine.
The student fumbles, she clamps and cuts the cord, blood is sprayed everywhere. She looks down at the baby and says 'It's a little girl.' There are screams of delight. The baby is wiped and dried and handed to the new mother.
The tension subsides as the new mother looks at the baby, the student wipes her forehead with her forearm and sighs. She prepares to deliver the placenta. The atmosphere in the delivery room changes. The midwives look more relaxed, almost at once all activity is focused on routines. The baby has to be labelled, washed, weighed. The second midwife begins to tidy away equipment. There is now a new set of seemingly important tasks to be completed.
'Let's get on' says the midwife.

Birth has much to do with emotional labour and is often about the intense professional–client interaction described by Hearn (1987). The business of birth is what the female semi-professionals can do when, as explained in Chapter 2, the doctor is absent and remote leaving the midwives doing the subordinated 'women's work'. It was clear that completing tasks such as 'doing the baby', 'doing the notes' was valued more highly by some, than the doing of 'emotional work'. There was an urgency to 'get on' and complete the real or proper work whilst the emotional labour or women's work seemed to assume a lesser importance.

The field-note extract presented above also illustrates the use of ritualistic phrases and expressions commonly used in midwifery. They are phrases which 'insiders' know well and which newcomers adopt quickly to become accepted members of the culture. Few outsiders would be familiar with the phrase 'she's fully' or the concept of 'wasting pains' or understand the significance of the phrase . . . 'Don't push, pant, pant, pant.' Many writers have demonstrated that communication within a hospital setting is frequently inadequate. Kirkham (1983) argues that the women she observed in her labour ward study wanted information with which to orientate themselves to their labours. Despite the efforts of the midwives she concluded that usually the information was inadequate. Women in labour have to rely on the midwife and their previous experience to interpret and understand the instructions they are given.

■ Sharing the work: real and unreal

Labour was often a prolonged lengthy affair with long periods of time when not much happened. The midwives explained that it was useful to have either a student or the woman's partner around as this person could stay with the woman. The Sisters explained (and I observed) that they rarely stayed with a woman throughout labour: the task was usually delegated to more junior staff midwives, student midwives and even student nurses. It was clear that for the sisters the real work was the birth itself and at all other times the midwife in charge would busy herself with administrative tasks, e.g. the ordering of drugs, equipment, stationery, etc. as well as answering the telephone and dealing with enquiries and the off-duty rota.

Another interesting phenomenon observed was the way in which the work was allocated. It appeared that at the start of a shift the complicated and potentially abnormal cases would be allocated to the most junior and newly qualified midwives. The women who appeared to be more likely to have a normal birth would be allocated to the sisters, although not the one in charge, and to a student midwife. When I asked questions to confirm my ideas the Sister explained that the student midwives needed 'cases' and needed to be supervised by experienced midwives whilst the newly qualified midwives needed experience. When I discussed this with the junior staff midwives they explained that they found the organisation of work very stressful. This is explored further in stresses and strains. They explained that life as a student midwife was more fun as they had more freedom to be involved in normal birth. Qualification was seen as a somewhat retrograde step where work on the labour ward meant long shifts looking after women in prolonged labour who usually ended up having either a forceps delivery or a Caesarian Section. It was clear that all midwives, whether newly qualified or experienced, saw their involvement with normal birth to be the most satisfying aspect of their job.

This is illustrated in Field note 5.5.

The delivery was clearly the most important aspect of labour ward work. When a delivery was imminent the staff would gather around outside the delivery room. Many midwives to whom I spoke, told me that they considered the birth to be the most important and vital aspect of the work. They said 'Well, if we get the delivery wrong, we have a dead baby, – that cannot be put right.' It was clear that this was the 'high spot' in their work. They would complain if, at the end of a shift, there had not been a birth. One midwife said, as she went off duty: 'Nothing much happened today. Only problems and nigglers. I haven't had a delivery all day.' A shift without a delivery was clearly not as rewarding as a shift with a delivery. To midwives it seems that birth matters most.

FN 5.5 _____

I arrived at the Hospital at 10a.m. It was very busy with women in advanced labour in each of the first stage and delivery rooms. There was a staff midwife in the office, whom I had not met before. She asked me who I was and if I was the new paediatric SHO. I gave my standard explanation which she accepted. She told me that she usually worked in the antenatal clinic where the hours were 'better'. She said she had small children and the regular clinic hours suited best. She went on to explain how she loved it when she was called to the labour ward. If it was very busy the midwives working in the antenatal clinic would come to the labour ward to help out. She then explained how it was quite difficult to get to know a woman who was sedated and in advanced labour but she coped. She didn't comment on how the woman coped. She explained with enthusiasm that work in clinic was alright but to be called to the labour ward to deliver a baby was 'the best bit of all'.

■ Rubber gloves and bloody arms

This section begins by considering some of the routines used to limit the spread of infection and how these routines reflected the staff's imperfect knowledge of the process of contagion. It also considers the attitudes of the staff to 'dirt' and its eradication.

Hospitals have been traditionally represented as clean places although the reality is, as we have seen, highly debatable. Disinfectants are sold to the householder, for example, urging the purchaser to make his or her home 'hospital clean'. In practice, hospitals are far from clean. Women who have recently given birth to a baby, and newborn babies, are particularly vulnerable to infection, so there is some justification in going to some lengths to ensure cleanliness. The delivery of a baby is not, in normal circumstances, a surgical procedure requiring operating-theatre standards of hygiene. Some progress in humanising the process has been made, in that partners are no longer required to don a mask, cap and gown to observe their child being born. Plastic aprons take the place of gowns but rubber gloves are still used extensively.

At the time of my research recent information and media panic on the subject of AIDS had resulted in an increased use of surgical rubber gloves. During the field work at Valley Maternity Unit after a baby had been born, all the equipment used was cleaned with hot water to remove blood, mucous, faeces, obstetric lubricating cream, etc., and then the equipment was wiped over with a disinfectant containing a high concentration of alcohol spirit.

Roth (1978) describes in his paper 'Ritual and Magic in the Control of Contagion' the uncertainties associated with the transmission of the disease of tuberculosis. He explained how these uncertainties resulted in ritualised procedures that depended more on convenience and ease of administration, than on rationally deduced probabilities.

Uncertainties about the mode of spread of the AIDS virus and the effect of this moral panic have produced similar ritualised procedures.

It was clear that most of the staff felt particularly vulnerable. They commented on how they came into contact with all types of body fluids and had no idea who was HIV positive and therefore infectious, and who was not. They responded to this fear by wearing gloves for most of the time. Field note 5.6 illustrates this further.

It would appear from these examples that many of the staff had no clear idea of when it was appropriate to wear gloves and when it was not. It has always been the practice in maternity hospitals to wear gloves for vaginal examinations and delivering the baby. Sometimes household rubber gloves would be provided and worn for general cleaning.

More recently the staff at Valley Maternity Unit had changed their practice in order to protect themselves against infection with AIDS virus or the Hepatitis B infection. They wore gloves most of the time, presumably in the hope that this would protect them from contamination. The surgical gloves which had replaced the household gloves, for routine cleaning and which were worn for all sorts of activities, seemed to have taken on an imagined 'magical' protective quality.

Nick Fox (1992:25) deconstructs the meaning of surgical sterilising procedures in an operating theatre in a similar manner.

FN 5.6

I was waiting in the reception area when a domestic assistant wearing rubber surgical gloves approached me. 'Can I help you' she said. She directed me to Mrs P.'s office and as I looked behind me she went into a little cupboard and still wearing her gloves proceeded to drink tea and smoke a cigarette.

I was amused to note that the nursing auxiliary was wearing rubber surgical gloves for her duties. She explained that all staff had been advised to wear gloves for cleaning as they may come into contact with blood and thus risk infection with AIDS or Hepatitis B. I was amused because she was wearing her gloves and apron to make and drink tea.

Sister (to staff midwife) 'We had better order more gloves. I always wear them on the job these days. You never know do you?'

Today I met a new student midwife on the labour ward, she was hot and tired, she told me she had just completed a delivery. She was writing the details of the case in the delivery book. When she had finished, still wearing rubber gloves, she opened the cupboard and prepared an injection of vitamin K for the baby.

■ Dirt and blood in midwifery practice

Labour ward work was certainly 'dirty'. A considerable amount of time was spent on cleaning equipment and delivery rooms, yet there was very little evidence in everyday practice of revulsion towards the dirt. On one occasion, two midwives were obliged to empty a rubbish bag on to the floor to search for a missing pair of forceps. Here, their attitude to dirt was totally different. They wore gloves and face-masks. They poked at the swabs and paper towels with a pair of long-handled forceps until they found the missing pair. Then they bundled the contents back into the bag, removed their gloves and masks, and rigorously washed and scrubbed their hands and arms.

Douglas (1976) in her extensive work 'Purity and Danger' describes dirt as 'matter out of place' and a threat to good order. Blood, swabs and debris on a trolley after a birth were not regarded as 'dirt', neither was blood on instruments, or on trolley wheels, in buckets or for that matter on arms or aprons. However, once delivery-room debris was placed in a plastic bin liner its identity appeared to change. It was now considered as 'dirt', 'matter out of place' and a threat to good order. If a midwife had to return to a rubbish bin and empty the contents on the floor its contents were viewed as dirt. A mask, gloves and distancing forceps were needed to deal with it.

The concept of dirt as 'matter out of place' can be expanded further by reference to Field note 5.7. This example illustrates the attitude of the midwives towards 'blood'. Although blood is generally regarded with some disdain, as a bodily fluid appropriate only in veins or in sealed specimen bottles, the midwives working on the labour ward seemed to attach greater importance to its presence on their person.

FN 5.7

I walked into the office with Mrs P. She introduced me to the Sisters and told them that I was a midwife doing some research. I noticed that, unlike the staff downstairs, no one was wearing a hat but all wore plastic aprons. I noticed that both Sisters wore aprons that were really quite dirty and covered with bloodstains. I also observed that both Sisters had bloodstains on their forearms. I must have looked for a little too long. Mrs P. glanced at their arms and said 'Busy morning, Sisters.' She smiled. 'Oh yes' they retorted, 'it has been really hectic.' They looked carefully at their arms and aprons and smiled proudly.

These bloodstains seemed to be acceptable. The senior midwife who was escorting me to the labour ward did not seem concerned about this apparent lack of cleanliness. The smile after her comment could be taken to mean that they were proud, not only of the blood on their arms, but of their morning's work. The question must be posed as to why blood was acceptable as a badge of battle or achievement at a time when there was such a fear of contracting HIV.

■ Unacceptable dirt

The final section considers, again, attitudes to dirt. Field note 5.8 was recorded as usual shortly after the incident observed. It was in the early evening when a woman arrived at the office door.

FN 5.8

There was a knock at the office door. The door was open and we saw a woman standing at the door. She was dressed in a thin dress and open soft shoes. It was a very cold evening. Her feet and clothes were very dirty and there was a distinctive unpleasant odour emanating from her person. She was with a man, untidily dressed and equally 'smelly'. The man stood silently as the woman dropped her head and began breathing deeply and slowly. The Sister moved towards them and asked if they has telephoned to arrange admission. They had not.

Sister said: 'You had better come this way' and directed the couple towards the admission room; then she turned back towards me. She held her nose and gesticulated, indicating that the woman had an offensive body odour.

When they arrived at the admission room the usual series of questions was directed at the woman, Mrs D. 'First Baby?' 'What's been happening?' etc. The Sister said: 'Well you need to go into the bath next, in there' (she pointed towards the bathroom) 'Have a good soak. You had better have a gown. Babies have to come to a clean area.' Sister returned to the office, and said to no one in particular 'God, that woman stinks. Soap and water are free – they are just lazy.'

I subsequently discovered that the couple had been living in a garage for some weeks, a fact publicised by a local paper. When Mrs D. emerged from the bathroom she was obviously in some considerable pain. The midwife helped her on to the bed and explained that she wanted to listen to the heart-beat. Her attitude towards the woman, now she was clean, was pleasant and helpful. Her partner was directed to a chair near her bed, he had not bathed, but was allowed complete with 'dirt', into the labour ward.

This extract illustrates how the staff view cleanliness and dirt. There is clearly a wish not to be too closely associated with substances that exude from the body. Most women who present themselves for admission to the labour ward have clearly recently bathed and are wearing clean underwear. Mrs D. however, was dirty. She was wearing old, dirty and inappropriate clothes. She was in labour, in pain, and in need of the help and support of a midwife. Yet she was treated as a deviant. She was dirty and had not telephoned to arrange admission. She was instructed to go to the bathroom, even though this might not have been the most appropriate course of action for someone in advanced labour. The midwife distanced herself from her physically and emotionally until she was clean. A final comment was very helpful, as the woman moved into the bathroom the midwife said to me 'It's a pity there are no students on tonight.' I asked why and she explained that she would have sent a student to escort the woman and perhaps supervise her bath. Her comment and explanation confirmed what many of the students had said. That is, that as students they are often treated as a pair of hands and allocated menial tasks. I did not consider that supporting this woman was a menial task but clearly it was considered inappropriate for a qualified midwife to be involved in the removal of dirt.

■ Criteria for moral evaluation of women and their partners

Kelly and May (1982) writing in the *Journal of Advanced Nursing* present an extensive critique of the literature of 'good' and 'bad' patients. They found that patients with certain illnesses, diseases and symptoms were more or less popular with doctors and nurses. It was also reported that popularity depended on age, gender, race and class characteristics. The midwives at Valley Maternity Hospital appeared to use a variety of criteria to conduct moral evaluations of the clientele. It was clear from analysis of the field notes that the major consideration in assessing a woman's worth was in the assessment of her status as a 'niggler' or a 'labourer'. This is explored more fully in Chapter 6. However, there was other evidence of 'moral' evaluation.

Social class was an important aspect. The midwives explained to me that the first thing they did when they obtained the notes of a woman expected to arrive in labour was to look at the occupation of her partner and herself. They explained that they were comfortable knowing in advance if they were dealing with the partner of a company director, a salesman, a bricklayer or, most commonly, the unemployed. They explained that it seemed that most men in the area were unemployed, although this was not in fact true. They explained 'I always look at the notes. You are bound to speak differently to the posh than to the unemployed.' Having been given the cue, I carefully watched to see if the communication differed from their description. It seemed that those who were in social class I and II (as defined by the occupation of the male head of the household) had more lengthy communications and more detailed explanations. Women whose partners were in the lower social classes had a more standard type of communication. As Stimpson and Webb (1975) have shown this professional adjustment to the social class of a client is part of the interaction process.

It also appeared that the midwives assessed women according to their language and social competencies. Women who were school teachers were labelled as 'knowing too much' and having 'read too many books' and frequently the comment was made that an abnormal labour with some intervention was more likely for these women.

As part of the admission routine the midwife would unpack the suitcase and it was during this procedure that the midwife would often make an assessment of the woman's social position. Field note 5.9 gives one midwife's explanation.

FN 5.9

You can tell what type they are by their case. Do they shop at Marks and Spencer or Primark? Do they not shop at all? Some come in with dirty clothes and a carrier bag. I call that laziness. They have money for fags and then wear old clothes.

Women's age was another important feature. There was obvious evidence of ageism. Women over 30 were handled with greater caution despite the fact that the literature advises that the increased risk in childbirth to women over 30 is greatly exaggerated.

Body size was also an important feature of the moral evaluation. Obese women were considered to be in some way 'out of control' having 'let themselves go' and always totally responsible for their size. The comments recorded in Field note 5.10 reflect this. Some comments were made in the women's presence and sometimes out of earshot in the office or corridor.

FN 5.10

Midwife (to woman): 'Get on to the couch, if you can – We haven't got a hoist.'

'Someone is going on a diet when this lot is over.'

Midwife (as she palpates a woman's abdomen) 'There is a baby in there somewhere, underneath this eiderdown'.

'I'll have to have help with *these* legs.'

'God knows if they can do an epidural through that lot.'

'She is huge and she is a teacher.'

'Been eating for two have you?'

The next aspects of moral evaluation related to personal hygiene. A detailed example of this evaluation is described earlier in this chapter in 'Rubber Gloves and Bloody Arms'. There were many examples in the field notes where the midwives are recorded as commenting openly about aspects of personal hygiene. Field note 5.11 gives some.

FN 5.11

'Have you seen the colour of her feet, she can't have washed them for months.'

'I'm not examining Mrs C. until she's been in the bath'.

'Have these pants been washed?' (Holding up a discoloured pair of the woman's undergarments)

'Have you seen her husband's shirt? He must have worn that one down the pit.'

The intellect of both women and their partners was frequently discussed and comment was openly made when a woman was considered to be of limited ability. Various euphemisms were used and recorded. Field note 5.12 gives some examples.

FN 5.12

'She is two sandwiches short of a picnic.'

'Short on grey cells'

'Her brain is in her feet.'

'Not much upstairs.'

'Thick as a brick.'

'Thick as two short planks.'

'She doesn't know how she got pregnant!'

'Not a University graduate'

'They seem to have the ability to get in to this state but not to get out of it.'

■ You can't trust a mother

Another theme that emerged during the study reflected the attitudes of some midwives towards some women in their care. There are often lessons to be learnt from describing good practice and examples are included throughout the book. The midwives were kind, warm and compassionate human beings who were generally able to communicate very well with women. Examples of good practice were observed and enjoyed and reported as part of the study. It may be that the emphasis of this study seems to focus on aspects of bad or at least less than good practice and why this may be so is discussed in Chapter 3. My position was to be an outsider on the inside or a 'marginal native', poised between stranger and friend. The good practice that I observed became part of me as 'an insider' enjoying my profession and good midwifery care. On reflection it would have been a better ethnography if more examples of good midwifery care had been included.

Ethnography searches for meanings, it looks for themes and seeks examples. The evidence presented in this section is here as part of the ethnography of a labour ward. I hope that it will encourage some midwives to question their practice and reconsider their assumptions. The title of this section 'You can't trust a mother' is a direct quote from the field notes and examples that seem to support this somewhat distrustful attitude are presented.

The first example describes a common event observed during the study. The labour ward telephone rang and I assumed the other side of the conversation, which followed these lines.

Caller: I think I might be pregnant.
Midwife: Hello, what was that? You think you might be pregnant? You need a GP not the labour ward.

I could not help feeling rather sad that the midwife had nothing to offer this woman, who had summoned the courage to ring her local maternity unit.

The next frequently observed phone call went something like this:

Caller: Hello . . . I think I am in labour. I've been having pains since last Tuesday, the pains went away on Wednesday, but well they're back now . . . coming every five minutes.
Midwife: Well you had better come in now so that *we* can decide!!!

I observed the midwife to be taking control: 'Come in and we will decide'.

Field note 5.13 gives other examples that illustrate how the midwives disregard, or disbelieve what women say.

These examples illustrate how some midwives systematically disempowered women at all stages in the childbirth experience. Women's opinions, previous knowledge and experience were devalued by the so-called experts. Frequently it was because the midwives practised using a medical model of care. They were conditioned into believing that pregnant women, like other people who entered hospital, were ill and must have decisions taken out of their hands. Unconsciously they removed from women the right to be in control of their own bodies.

FN 5.13

Woman:	I'm having terrible contractions, they are really strong.
Midwife:	Feel quite weak to me.

Woman:	I feel that the head has gone down – it's much easier to breathe, I feel more comfortable.
Midwife:	Um, yes well it's still three-fifths.

['three-fifths' means that three-fifths of the head can still be felt via the abdomen and birth is still some time away.]

Woman:	I think my waters must have gone. (Standing in a pool of water).
Midwife:	Just 'pop' on the couch and I will test with one of these sticks.

Woman:	I don't want anything for pain just now – I seem to be doing alright.
Midwife:	They're going to get much worse you know – you would be better to have Pethidine now.

Woman:	I think I want to push.
Midwife:	You can't do . . . I have only just examined you.

Woman:	I must get up and go to the toilet. I want to open my bowels.
Midwife:	It's only the baby's head pressing down.

Woman:	I want my partner here all the time.
Midwife:	I am sending him for some tea . . . he needs a rest.

Woman:	I would like my small children to be present for the delivery.
Midwife:	Oh, I really don't think you should . . . it's not very nice, too hot and all that blood!

Woman:	I don't want to breast-feed the baby.
Midwife:	Are you sure? It's really best for babies, you know.

Woman:	My baby is due this week.
Midwife:	What date did we give you? You must have had a scan.

Presented in this fashion it might appear to the reader that the midwives at Valley Maternity Hospital were arrogant, self-opinionated and totally judgemental. This would be unfair and untrue. There were very many occasions when the midwives gave care that was kind, intelligent, sensitive and totally unconditional. However, it is important to ask why some midwives needed to express themselves in this way and why the researcher appeared to focus on aspects of bad practice. There were many examples of good practice and as explained in Chapter 3 to be a midwife and a researcher was not always easy.

It is still worth asking why this female workforce needed to assert their superiority over the women in their care. As has been argued in Chapter 2, it seems that the acquired knowledge of the professional woman (the midwife) has to be seen to dominate the experiential knowledge of the 'natural woman' (the mother).

Chapter 6

Organisation and control

■ **Getting through the work**

The phrase 'getting through the work' was coined by Clarke (1978) who, in a paper of the same name, sought to discover the meanings that nurses attached to their work. She was particularly interested in definitions of work and the implications of those definitions for subsequent changes in working practices.

I was interested in the midwives' definition of 'work' and this section considers how the midwives at Valley Maternity Hospital 'get through the work'. The chapter includes a description of the ways in which two types of admission were dealt with by the midwives. These categories of admission I have called 'the labourers' and 'the nigglers'.

During the course of my fieldwork I observed a series of conversations between midwives, when they discussed the difficulties they experienced in diagnosing accurately the onset of labour. They commented on the fact that although midwifery textbooks listed the various criteria, in practice there were often difficulties in diagnosis. They described how the latent or early stages of labour could vary in length from one to two hours, to a matter of days and said that, if, on arrival, a woman was found to be in the active phase of labour, i.e. the cervix or neck of the womb had opened to, say, 4 of the required 10 centimetres and she was having strong regular contractions, there would be no problems and she would be admitted. Another midwife involved in this discussion explained that if she knew that a woman was in active labour it was safe to assume that she would probably give birth within a reasonable amount of time and as such would not 'block' a labour ward bed.

The midwives explained to me how important it was to keep some delivery beds free, so that appropriate facilities were available for those in advanced labour. Some women arrived and gave birth to their baby in a very short space of time. These women could not wait for a bed to become available.

A woman admitted in established labour was usually taken to the delivery room. One of the midwives made an interesting comment about this, which is recorded in the field notes:

'They come in and we offer them a choice – it's a joke really, the choice only exists to '4 centimetres', then they are in bed and slapped on a monitor. It's best if they don't come in until they are further on really. You know, if they want a more natural birth.'

This comment is interesting because the midwife was describing those aspects of labour ward work that she disliked. The staff were aware of the consumer criticism, and felt that they were only paying lip-service to consumer demands, e.g. the Active Birth Movement attaches a great deal of importance to mobility in labour. Many books, e.g. Balaskas (1983), explain that labour is less painful and likely to be shorter if women are not confined to bed. At Valley Maternity Hospital the procedure dictated by the consultant obstetricians, insisted that every woman in labour had the fetal heart rate and contraction frequency monitored for most of the labour. This meant that the woman had to be in bed whilst a transducer was attached with straps to her abdomen. The Sister's comment reflected her distaste for this routine practice. She felt that the only way of avoiding this style of management was for the woman to arrive at the labour ward well-advanced in labour or (it transpired later) at night.

Sudnow (1967) in his book, *Passing On*, said that dying was essentially a predictive term and it was possible to tell that someone was dying just by looking at them. There was a set of observable happenings that informed the observer that death would occur in a specific time. Sudnow described dying as a series of 'organisationally relevant events'. He described how on one occasion a young doctor incorrectly predicted the time of death. The family made extensive preparations with resultant severe embarrassment for the doctor involved.

Similarly, in labour, there is a set of observable known-about or assumed happenings which tell the midwife that labour and subsequently, delivery, will occur in a predictable number of hours. The midwives rely on these phenomena to control the workload of the unit, but sometimes the signs fail the observer.

The midwives relied on various signs to inform them of the rate of progress of labour. They conducted vaginal examinations and were able to predict by the dilatation and consistency of the cervix, the rate at which it was likely to dilate and when the baby would be born. They also developed with experience a 'gut feeling' and almost intuitively knew when birth is imminent. A midwife was observed merely looking at a woman and commenting 'Oh she is cracking on – it won't be long.'

It was important to make fairly accurate predictions about the time of birth. Relatives anxiously enquired and often the woman's partner needed to have a good idea of the likely time scale in order to make his domestic arrangements. If the midwife miscalculated the relatives might lose faith in her judgement and in her clinical expertise. She may also find that she has a woman who is blocking a labour ward for too long. Sudnow describes a problem that is eventually resolved, in his study the patient dies. In the labour ward, the resolution of the problem, i.e. delivering the baby, may utilise all the available staff for a prolonged period. This is why it was important as far as possible to 'get it right' and make an accurate prediction.

It is now proposed to develop these two themes further predicting the time of birth and organising the through-put of work on the labour ward.

The midwife's main aim, when she started a shift, was only to admit to the delivery suite, those who were definitely in labour, and then 'get them delivered' and transferred to the post-natal wards, as soon as possible. It was the usual practice for women to be moved from the delivery room to the post-natal ward within one and a half hours of the baby being born. This way the labour ward beds could be kept free. As previously explained, some women would arrive without warning and require a delivery room as a matter of urgency. This fact represents a continual pressure on the midwife in charge who must always have accommodation available to meet this contingency.

■ The nigglers and the labourers

Women who presented themselves in labour were classified by the midwives in the following way:

(a) The *'labourers'*, who were in established labour and for whom admission was readily justified.
(b) The *'nigglers'*, who were often described as 'not doing much'. These women were in the early stages of labour. This stage varies in length from two or three hours to two or three days.

'Labourers' were women who arrived well-advanced in labour. They were welcomed by the midwife as 'real work'. Their admission was justified, they would be delivered of their baby in a reasonable amount of time and would not block a labour ward bed. Admissions of this nature were viewed favourably by midwives and student midwives who were anxious to 'get a case'.

At the time of the admission, the procedure described in Chapter 5 would take place. The midwife would make an assessment and then make the decision to allocate the women to the labour ward, 'niggling room' or antenatal ward. A wrong decision would result in a blocked bed or a rapid unplanned return to the labour ward.

■ Guessing and assessing

□ The labourers

During the course of the fieldwork I noted a series of conversations between midwives. It became clear that there were difficulties in accurately diagnosing the onset of labour. Even if the midwives followed the 'letter of the law' some women would surprise them. The midwives argued that it was important to keep some beds free so that appropriate facilities would be available for those arriving in advanced labour. Thus it appeared that the midwife's main aim when she started a shift was only to admit to the delivery suite those women who were definitely in labour. Her subsequent aim was to 'get them delivered' and transferred to the post-natal ward as soon as possible. Labourers – the real work on the delivery suite – were women who arrived in established labour. Their admission was justified, they would deliver in a reasonable time and would not block a bed. Labourers were also welcomed by student midwives who were anxious for further experience. Nigglers, as stated, were often described as 'not doing much'. These women were in the early stages of labour, often they had backache, some had contractions. Field note 6.2 illustrates these points.

The first example reports a conversation between a student midwife and a Sister, where they discuss a Mrs S, who as a 'niggler' had been transferred to the antenatal ward earlier in the day.

FN 6.2

Student: That Mrs S we sent to the ward this morning – they are sending her back. Is that OK?

Sister: Yes, they don't like them to have Pethidine on the antenatal ward.

Student: Um, so well, they come here if they need analgesia then? Does that mean it doesn't matter about the cervix then, just if she needs Pethidine?

Sister: (Sighs) No, it's not as simple as that, it's all assessed individually. We decide if they need Pethidine. If they are 'distressed' we would admit them. If they are not then they don't need it, and anyway we are not allowed to give it if they are not in labour. Anyway, if they are okay at home or on the wards we don't admit them unless the pains are too much for them or they are making a lot of fuss. We can't have the place cluttered up by women who are not really in labour.

Re-admission was permitted because in this case Mrs S. was 'distressed' or perhaps making 'a lot of fuss' or simply that she required intramuscular analgesia.

Field notes 6.3 and 6.4, drawn directly from the field notes, demonstrate how the midwife in charge is the 'lynch pin', and how she attempts to control the flow of 'work'. The examples illustrates how the doctors were aware of the constraints of the system and accepted arrangements which meant a delay in obstetric interventions. In each case I wrote up the conversations in the field notes on the same evening.

FN 6.3

Sister (to student): You see, you have to learn to keep the doctors under control. It's up to us to decide who we will admit and who we won't. They think they decide, but well – we can't refuse anyone, but well, we can control the timing. I mean you can't give good care to too many. What is the point of inducing someone when the labour ward is hectic. An induction is more risky than a normal case. You don't go inviting trouble do you? You see, it's far better that we get this lot delivered and shipped off to the wards before we accept any more. Anyway (she laughed) I'm a much nicer midwife if I've had a cup of tea, so put the kettle on.

FN 6.4

There was one Sister and two staff midwives on duty. They had had a busy morning, with four babies being born all within a short space of time. When I arrived, the Sister was in the office, checking drugs and the midwives were in the sluice room, chatting as they washed down the trolleys. The newly delivered mothers were all in various stages of preparation for transfer to the wards. The phone rang; from one side of the conversation I gathered that on the antenatal ward there was a woman, who, though not in established labour, required admission and acceleration of labour for an obstetric complication. The woman was a 'niggler' but could easily have become a 'labourer'.

The Sister made her decision and said: 'Oh, we have been hectic, the place is a tip, we haven't cleared the decks yet. Give us an hour or so to get straight'.

I presumed that the person on the other end of the phone consented to this arrangement. Sister wandered out and said to the staff midwife 'They wanted to do an ARM (artificial rupture of the membranes). I've told them to wait until after lunch.'

'Thank God for that', she said, 'I'll be off at 2.30. I'm shattered.'

On another occasion, a staff midwife was observed to be putting pressure on a doctor to act on a case, because the unit was quiet and the staff felt able to cope. The case concerns a Mrs C who was in early labour and it is recorded in Field note 6.5.

FN 6.5

Mrs C is a Gravida 5 and a known drug-user. It is believed that she has previously been infected with the Hepatitis B virus. The staff are somewhat confused as to how this case should be managed, so as to avoid risks of cross-infection. Mrs C has come into hospital with 'weak contractions and ruptured membranes'.

The staff midwife, basing her argument on Mrs C.'s history wants 'to get her delivered'. She argues that with Syntocinon her labour will be induced quickly and that as the unit is quiet, it is a good time to 'start her off'. The doctor is reluctant. He is due in theatre at 8.00 p.m. and wants to eat before he goes. The doctor rings his senior to discuss the case. He is dismissive of what the midwife has described as 'weak niggling contractions'. He convinces his senior that the best management is to transfer to another ward to 'await events'. The decision made, he firmly closes the case notes and goes for a meal. The woman is transferred to the ward.

Here the midwife tried to exert her influence on the management of a case. Her priority was to 'get her [the woman] delivered'. The unit was quiet and she felt that it was a good time to start a potentially complicated case (i.e. a known drug-user, Hepatitis B infected, an induced labour).

The doctor concerned, who would be responsible for actually inducing labour, had other things on his mind, his planned visit to the operating theatre and the need to have his supper. In this case the midwife did not successfully exert her control over the labour ward and her work, but had a good try.

☐ **The 'nigglers'**

The 'nigglers' were dealt with in three ways. If the labour ward was quiet labour might be induced. If the midwives were uncertain of the diagnosis, the woman might spend some time in the 'niggling room'. If the labour ward was busy, the woman would almost invariably be transferred to the antenatal ward to 'await events'. The field notes illustrate this typology.

On one occasion when the unit was not unduly busy a woman arrived by ambulance. She was in the early stages of labour and would normally have been designated a 'niggler'. However, on this occasion, the labour ward was quiet and a student midwife who needed the experience of deliveries was on duty. The case was managed for the benefit of the student. Field note 6.6 tells the story.

On other occasions 'nigglers' would be treated in a different fashion. They were generally regarded as an irritation to the staff, who felt that admitting a 'niggler' was time-consuming work with no end-result. The admission procedure involved all the routines described in Chapter 5 as well as a period of continuous monitoring. Field note 6.7 illustrates this point.

FN 6.6

Sister was reading Mrs P.'s notes. Mrs P. had telephoned to say that she was having contractions and was coming in. Sister noted that this was her third pregnancy and pointed out to the student midwife that Mrs P. had two previously normal deliveries following relatively short labours of eight and six hours respectively. She flipped through the notes and said: 'This one looks hopeful for you. You are on until 9 (it was 4.00 p.m.) so you should be okay.'

The woman, Mrs P., was duly admitted. Later the student midwife conducted a vaginal examination and was encouraged by the Sister to augment the progress of labour by rupturing the membranes. Mrs P. did indeed deliver by 8.30 p.m. The student had the case and Mrs P her baby.

FN 6.7

Mrs B. had arrived at the hospital with her mother, her sister, and some way behind, her reluctant partner. It was her first baby and her third admission in this pregnancy, supposedly in labour. Mrs B. was very anxious that this admission would not be another false alarm. She said that she was sorry to cause so much trouble but the pains were really strong at home, but always seemed to go away once she and her family had arrived at the hospital.

Mrs B. was whisked away into the admission room. I did not have an opportunity to seek her consent to observe, so stayed outside. Within minutes the Sister emerged and shouted across the corridor to the office to the other Sister, '2 cms – not doing much, needs a run then we will ship her off to the wards.'

A 'run' is a period of monitoring the heart beat of the fetus, and any contractions. It usually takes about twenty minutes. The midwife does not normally stay with the woman but is still responsible for her care until she is transferred to the antenatal ward.

The Sister in this case was openly hostile to Mrs B. She complained in the office to her colleagues that 'if only these women went to classes, they would know when to come in'. This was not strictly true but illustrated the midwife's frustration at having to spend time on non-productive work.

Sometimes if the midwife was not sure if the woman was a niggler or a labourer, she would arrange for her to spend some time in the 'niggling room'. This was a small room with four beds, situated close to the labour ward. It was run and staffed by the labour ward staff.

On one occasion, after a busy morning, the 'niggling room' was occupied by three women who had arrived in labour, but who had not yet progressed to established labour. The nursing auxiliary walked into the office and said 'Shall I ship this lot down to the wards? They make the place look untidy.'

Nigglers were viewed as an intrusion into a busy labour ward; they presented the staff with a problem and were readily categorised as 'bad' patients. Good patients were those who, by presenting themselves in established labour allowed the midwives to do their job 'properly', according to their definition.

Jeffrey (1979) describes how patients visiting casualty departments, were typified as 'good' or 'bad'. The staff attempted to deter 'bad' patients from returning by making their experience as uncomfortable as possible. In the labour ward setting the woman will inevitably return. The midwives, though rarely hostile, expressed their frustration with 'bad patients' out of earshot.

Roth (1972) and Strong and Davis (1978) describe the moral evaluation of patients in various medical meetings and Murcott (1981) states that 'Patients are identified as "bad" or otherwise by staff in judging events, resources, objects and people in the course of a working day.' She believes that this typification is a normal feature of medical settings. She goes on to describe how sociological accounts of medical work report that a wide range of criteria are used for the moral evaluation of clients. She lists such aspects as social class, social competencies, age, sex, body-size and personal hygiene, marital status and failure to adapt to ward routine. This issue is explored in more detail in Chapter 5.

It would seem that in a labour ward setting, the morality of an admission is related to the dilatation of the cervix. As Mrs B. said to me, after her vaginal examination 'Oh dear, when is it going to happen? When will I go into labour? I feel so responsible for the state of my cervix.'

■ Rules of admission

This chapter has presented evidence to support the list of unwritten rules that emerged during the fieldwork. It appeared that the rules of admission to the labour ward were as follows:

1. A 'niggler' who was sufficiently 'distressed' to require intramuscular Pethidine or someone who was making 'a lot of fuss' could be admitted. (NB: Administration of Pethidine does not necessarily confirm, indicate or guarantee the onset of labour.)
2. Admission for labour to be induced or accelerated was allowed but only if the midwife felt she could cope with the additional workload and had her tea. (The significance of tea is explained later.)
3. Complicated cases were encouraged if the labour ward was quiet.
4. 'Optimistic nigglers' could be considered for admission, i.e. those likely to deliver with minimal intervention, but only on those occasions when a student needed a case.

This chapter has considered how the midwives working at Valley Maternity Hospital 'get through' and exert control over their work. It has noted the midwives' frustration at not being able to offer the kind of care that the pressure groups and home-birth protagonists would want. It describes how in these circumstances there are good organisational and sociological reasons for organising the admissions in the way they do. It also considers the attitudes of the staff towards those women who are 'bad' or deviant because they are 'nigglers'.

The 'nigglers' were individuals who frustrated the midwives in their most productive role, that of a safe delivery of live, healthy babies. Nigglers were typified as 'bad patients' who failed because their cervix had not yet dilated.

■ Writing notes and drinking tea

As the fieldwork progressed it became clear that writing notes and drinking tea were frequently observed activities. The Valley Maternity Hospital was a very hot place with a temperature of around 24–26°C. No one ever complained of cold even in the depth of winter. The staff wore cotton dresses, some wore a belt and some chose to wear a paper nurse's cap although there was no clear policy on this. Some chose to wear theatre dress, which as previously described was a blue-and-green trouser suit. The labour ward was particularly hot, especially in the delivery room. It was clear that all the staff needed drinks at quite frequent intervals. Drinking tea appeared to carry more significance than merely the quenching of thirst. This section describes how tea-breaks were seen by the staff as a reward for a job well done. The tea-break was a legitimate opportunity to stop other work and finish writing-up the notes, whilst in the meantime imbibing numerous cups of tea. On the first occasion that I observed this aspect of labour ward culture, I made the following notes (Field note 6.8). There are many examples in the fieldwork notes that provide evidence of the activity described below.

After each delivery the mother and her companion were offered tea. The tea was made in the office and unless another delivery was imminent it was recognised as an opportunity or an excuse to stop and have an official break. These breaks made life on the labour ward more tolerable. The staff rewarded themselves before, after and sometimes between, each burst of activity. They provided an opportunity for the staff to recover physically and emotionally, and to share with their colleagues the events of birth. It was an opportunity for a cathartic release and airing of tension.

These tea-breaks, it would seem, were a normal part of labour ward culture. The ethnographer seeks meanings in the everyday activity and for midwives 'drinking tea' was unofficial therapy. It was the opportunity to unpack the experiences of being a midwife and to take and offer support to learners and colleagues.

FN 6.8

10.30 a.m. The office is in its usual untidy state – papers and half-eaten toast, cold tea are everywhere. The unit has been very busy – five babies have been born in the last hour. The staff explain that the shift system allows for two paid ten-minute tea-breaks, they feel this merely fulfils the letter of the law as laid down by the Health and Safety at Work Act and claim that it is always too busy to take official breaks. They justify regular and sometimes prolonged tea/toast and coffee-breaks by arguing that on many occasions they do not take their full entitlement of breaks.

The ashtrays are full and smoke pervades the air, though no one is currently smoking and all the staff appear to have been previously working. The Sister explains that she snatches a smoke when she can.

The staff, after a delivery, sit down at the table, sigh and complain of their exhaustion. They take an unofficial break while they 'write the notes'. They complain that it is not a 'real' break because they do not leave the delivery unit.

Smoking a cigarette, eating a piece of toast or a biscuit are the normal and usual types of behaviour. The 'rest' is justified by the rigours of the earlier session, a minimal reward for a job well done.

'Writing the notes' was another ritual undertaken after each birth. Each midwife had her own method of completing the forms and always followed the same order. The student midwives were taught 'the routine' by each midwife with whom they worked. Some would start at the beginning and work their way systematically from front to back. Others would always fill in the labour ward record-sheet first. The students often complained that the notes were more complicated to learn than the technique of delivering a baby. Apart from the notes themselves, there were additional forms to complete. These included:

(a) the birth notification form;
(b) pathology forms for cord blood samples;
(c) a neonatal discharge form;
(d) the Kardex or nursing record;
(e) Register of Births.
(f) the computer record of the birth

There was considerable repetition of information on the notes and corresponding forms and most midwives complained as they wrote. They said, for example, that they had to record the baby's weight in six places. If a delivery occurred at the changeover of shift (a situation which was avoided if at all possible) the midwife who was due off-duty would seek the assistance of her colleagues in completing the notes and would only complete those details which were her legal responsibility, e.g. Birth Register, notification and signature. Although the notes were generally viewed as being a chore, it was apparent that one must be a qualified midwife either to complete the notes or supervise their completion. This, then, became a prestigious task, allowing the midwife to sit down and drink tea, whilst they were completed.

It was also interesting that while the midwife was completing this task she was able quite legitimately to refuse to deliver other babies unless there was no one else free to attend to the women in labour. She might be called on to assist at another delivery but this was avoided if possible. During this period, i.e. while the midwife wrote the notes, the nursing auxiliary would wash the mother and baby, serve tea and arrange to transfer both parties to the post-natal ward. The bed was then washed and remade, the floor washed, and trolleys re-laid to await the next case.

It was also noted that the final stages of the task, i.e. the bed washing, was not completed until the auxiliary nurse had a 'break', and a quick unofficial cup of tea. On one occasion, as she poured the tea, the auxiliary said 'Isn't it marvellous how a mother loves a cup of tea after having a baby.' I agreed and noted that not only the woman, but also her partner, the midwife, the auxiliary nurse and sometimes the researcher, 'loved a cup of tea'. It was usual practice to make a large pot. The delivery rooms were even hotter than the office and corridor areas. On one occasion, after the delivery, the note-writing and the tea drinking were complete, I noted the following incident (see Field note 6.9).

FN 6.9

The Sister stood up, yawned and stretched. She adjusted her hat and her apron and then replaced her shoes. Turning to the student, she said 'Right, wheel 'em in, I'm ready for anything now.'

The Sister had written the notes, drunk her tea and completed her 'legal' period of abstaining from work.

It was also interesting to observe a new student midwife's introduction to the delivery suite. Here it was possible to deduce the importance that was attached to the tea-drinking. First, the student was carefully shown the open cupboard where she should store her handbag. (I noted that the staff trusted not only each other, but also everyone else who might enter the multipurpose office.) She was then shown where the tea, coffee, sugar and milk were stored. She was firmly encouraged to make tea whenever she wanted to and reminded that labour ward work was hot and busy work. The rules of the organisation and its cultural activities appeared clear.

Drinking tea and writing notes were major activities on the delivery suite. Ethnographic research looks for culturally embedded norms which guide the actions of individuals within a specific culture. During the period of my observations there was sufficient evidence to support the notion that it was the 'norm' to drink tea at frequent intervals whilst on the delivery suite.

The ethnographer can also speculate on these rituals and ask if there is any other significance in this apparent obsession with tea-drinking. It was certainly a physiological necessity to replace fluid, but it was also a mechanism for controlling the amount of work for which each midwife was responsible and a reward, self-administered for a job well done. Drinking tea was also the means by which the midwives relaxed and unwound after a birth.

The role of tea-drinking in the co-counselling process was also clear. Psychological support to students, colleagues and even junior house officers was offered during tea-drinking.

■ Aspects of communication

□ Verbal asepsis

Communication is an important feature of effective midwifery care. When it fails the woman can be dissatisfied or even damaged. There are examples throughout the book where communication was inadequate. In Chapter 5, 'Admissions', a woman was not told of the significance of the dilation of the cervix and in Chapter 3 another woman was alarmed when a midwife crashed into a delivery room and said 'My God, she is dipping.' There were many examples in the field notes which mirrored Mavis Kirkham's study 'Labouring in the Dark' (1983). There were examples of the use of the term 'distressed' with its value-added meaning, explored earlier in this chapter. There were also many examples of 'verbal asepsis' (Kitzinger, 1978; and Kirkham, 1989). The midwives frequently blocked conversations developing or gave answers that sterilised the communications. Frequently I noted that women apologised to their carers. They often told the doctor, called for a forceps delivery, that they were sorry to trouble him.

Field note 6.10 illustrates this.

There were of course occasions when midwives took the time to give good clear information. When I interviewed women many told me that they were very pleased with the care but I felt that their expectations were very low. When women were given full, detailed and careful explanations of events, progress and procedures, they were frequently very happy with their care.

There is little point in cataloguing numerous incidences of poor communication although it represented a key theme in the field notes and is discussed further in the final chapter. There is no doubt that when specific attention was given to improving both interpersonal and communication skills, care was improved.

FN 6.10

Woman:	How much longer will it be?
Midwife:	Not long now.
Woman:	My back really aches, is that normal?
Midwife:	Yes.
Woman:	What did that doctor mean when he said 'She'll probably need some help'?
Midwife:	Don't worry about that.
Woman:	What does he mean 'It's a bit small'?
Midwife:	Everything's fine.
Woman:	Why do you break the water? Is it safe?
Midwife:	Yes, just routine, don't worry.
Woman:	What was that injection for?
Midwife:	Help you relax.
Woman:	Why does everyone stare at the monitor? Is everything all right?
Midwife:	Everyone just does. Don't worry.
Woman:	When can I go home?
Midwife:	Later, I expect.
Doctor:	I am going to give you a hand to get this baby out.
Woman:	Thank you. I am sorry to bother you, I should have been able to do this myself.

It was clearly very difficult for women to communicate when distressed, in pain and in an alien environment with a midwife they had not previously met. The Valley Maternity Hospital was no exception. The midwives were skilled and able to establish a rapport with women fairly quickly. Their enthusiasm and energy compensated to some extent for the faults of the system that allowed women to give birth in a strange environment.

☐ **Spreading the news**

This section develops the theme of control as expressed through other aspects of communication. It examines how the telephone was used by midwives and relatives – the midwives to maintain their professional identity and to separate themselves from the clientele – and the relatives to spread the news of birth.

During the course of the observations that were made at the Valley Maternity Hospital, it was noted that various principles were used to regulate the manner in which the news of the birth and the progress of labour was spread to other members of the woman's family. It was noted that the telephone was also used by the 'organisation' to regulate the extent of the information being disseminated to enquirers.

It was possible to observe how, when, and to whom the news of a birth was made available. The maternity unit had a public call box available for relatives, it was surrounded, however, with notices that placed restrictions on its use, e.g. 'Do not use the phone at night', 'Not to be used by visitors', 'Not to be used by patients from other wards', etc.

The office, previously described, had a telephone and theoretically neither staff nor relatives were permitted to make outside calls. The hospital telephone handbook stated that the switchboard should be informed if a private call was to be made so that the person involved could be billed with the appropriate amount. This rule was observed to be broken very frequently. Indeed, I was aware that on one occasion I had probably 'gone native' when I asked the Sister-in-charge if I could ring home. She agreed without further comment. I was indeed an accepted part of the culture I was attempting to study.

When the staff were required to work beyond their normal finish time I observed a steady stream of staff ringing home to inform their families of the reason for delay. At night when the atmosphere on the unit was much more relaxed it was not unusual for 'new' fathers to be allowed into the office to ring their relatives. This did not seem to happen during the day. Sometimes spreading the news of birth was relatively easy. It was frequently noted that the woman in labour was accompanied by what seemed to be most of her extended family. It was moving to observe her partner emerge from the labour ward and announce the news with such phrases as in Field note 6.11!

FN 6.11

'She's 'ad it. It's a boy. You ought to see him, 'ands as big as shovels.'

'It's really great, aye! It's a boy.'

'It's a girl, it's a girl, it's a girl.'

'God, that was hard. It's not called labour for nothing. It's a little girl.'

On other occasions it was observed that the office phone would ring and new grandparents would be enquiring and anxious for news.

As previously noted, whilst the Sister was explaining policies and practices to the student I acquired the relevant information as in Field note 6.12.

FN 6.12

Sister to student midwife:
'When they ring up to enquire you have to be really careful. If you tell someone she has had a boy and that person knows before someone else in the family – then there is all hell to pay. Someone got the sex wrong once. The family were mad. They were going to sue. You see, its their news. I like to leave it up to them to spread it around.'

She then went on the explain that she usually gave a vague answer and would tell them that the husband/partner would be ringing shortly. I noted that it was usually the job of the husband or partner to inform the relatives.

On one occasion a young new father told his wife that he had told her parents first, whilst actually I had observed his first call was to his own Mum and Dad. He enjoyed being congratulated and told them they were the first to know. He then rang his wife's parents and said 'Lynda wanted you to be the first to know.' He did not actually say that they were not. He put the phone down, turned to me, winked and laughed. 'Least said, soonest mended'. I smiled and assured him I would not divulge the confidence.

■ Enquiries and interruptions

During the period of observation I also noted how the midwives responded to telephone enquirers about progress in labour. These enquirers were generally regarded as an irritation and time-consuming intrusion into the world of the labour ward. Enquiries tended to be dealt with quickly and politely but the attitude expressed was that the husband/partner was present and fully informed and that it was his responsibility to disseminate this information to the couples' relatives. For example, on one occasion, as the phone was replaced the Sister said, 'Tell her husband to get in touch with his family – they are driving me mad.'

There was a stock of phrases that could be used and if the midwife could avoid coming to the phone she would, prompting her assistant to make the appropriate comments, e.g:

> 'Coming on nicely.'
> 'Not delivered yet.'
> 'Only in early labour.'
> 'Everything's fine, no news yet.'
> 'Still in labour.'
> 'Doctor's with her now.'
> 'In labour, all is well.'

Again, it was easy to see that if the midwife took a prolonged period of time to answer telephone enquiries with detailed comments she would in some way be neglecting her other duties. Thus there are organisational reasons to 'deal with' telephone calls and proceed with other matters.

There was another aspect of telephone calls worthy of note and this is best illustrated by my field notes. They show how the midwife in charge of the care was unwilling to estimate the time of the arrival of the baby. As mentioned in Chapter 6 'Getting Through the Work', if the midwife makes an incorrect guess she risks losing the woman's – and her partner's – confidence in her clinical ability. It also illustrated a reluctance on the part of the professional to share her knowledge completely. By keeping something back, the midwife was less likely to weaken her professional stance and dilute her autonomy, as shown by Field note 6.13.

FN 6.13

Mrs B. is in established labour, her progress so far has been normal. To my eye, which is that of an experienced midwife, there is little doubt that the baby will be born within the hour. However, in response to frequent telephone calls from Mrs B.'s family the following comment is made: 'Babies come when they are ready. Mr B. will ring if there is any news.'

However, Mr B. who sits patiently in the delivery room is not, as far as I am aware, reassured that labour is going well and delivery is imminent.

In response to his direct question 'How much longer will it be?' he is told 'When the apple is ripe it will fall' and 'All in good time'. Simultaneously the staff make preparations for the imminent delivery. Sister, teaching the student the procedure, says in an authoritative voice: 'Turn on the heater, open the pack, check the cot.'

I reflected that there seemed a reluctance on the part of the midwife to commit herself to the family, as to a time limit for the remaining length of labour. Perhaps like the intern in Sudnow's ethnography of dying, the midwife was 'wary of premature proclamations'. Perhaps it was the conscious or unconscious desire to keep something back, or perhaps it was a symbol of her control of the events.

I understood the rationale of withholding information if it might mislead; grandparents may become irate if a long-awaited grandchild does not arrive when it is expected. However, I found it difficult to understand why the midwife chose to keep this information to herself. Here yet again I had great difficulty in separating professional judgement from ethnographic work. I was annoyed that the midwife did not take time to reassure and give information to the woman and her relatives. I wanted to take over the care. Instead I withdrew and wrote some notes in a private place.

This section has dealt with two important aspects of labour ward work. The first considered how information was exchanged between women and their families and the second looked at the way the midwives make use of the telephone. Field note 6.14 illustrates the feelings the midwives have, not only about the telephone and its use but also how closely they guard their professional knowledge. This conversation was recorded soon after the event and as far as I can remember is a verbatim account.

FN 6.14 _____

Sister to student midwife:
You see, the telephone on the labour ward is a blessing and a curse. Oh, of course we need to summon medical aid when we need it. And we have to be able to ring home when we are going to be late home for the fourth time this week; but in other ways it's a bit of a drag; the relatives they nag, nag, nag. They just ring up and say 'Has she had it?' 'Has who had what?' I reply. Then they say 'My sister, of course.' They don't give a name. Then when we tell them she hasn't had it, they want to know when! I always add a few hours on and tell them to ring back later. (She laughs heartily). A few hours later, when I have gone off duty! They seem to want to know everything these days. It's the telly I suppose. Some read too many books, that's for sure.'

Here we have an example of a midwife who resents the woman's relatives because they, in her opinion, prevent her from doing her job properly. Hughes (1971) has pointed out that a common complaint of people in the professions who perform a service for others is that they are somehow prevented from doing their duty as it should be done. In this example, the midwife feels that the telephone impinges upon her time and prevents her from getting on with the job of being a midwife.

This conversation also helps to describe the relationship between the midwife, as a professional and the woman as her client. Any personal-service professional has to exert some form of control over the client, so that she or he is not totally overwhelmed by their demands.

Chapter 7

Shifts and handovers

■ Continuity of care?

When this study began the main area of interest related to the theme of continuity of carer and the belief that the disruption in the care of women in labour was most acute when one midwife went off duty and handed over the care of the woman to another midwife. Total continuity of carer from pregnancy through labour and into the post-natal period seemed to be an impossibility or at least an unlikely pattern of care for most women.

Some researchers have argued that even to try to offer such care would be a retrograde step for the midwifery profession and for many midwives who have homes and families. Sandwell (1993) argues that the move for greater continuity and its emphasis on 'round-the-clock' care is also likely to penalise the army of midwives who currently work part-time.

Robinson *et al.* (1983) demonstrated that 46.8 per cent of midwives were willing to work flexible hours to provide continuity of care throughout labour and delivery. The remainder of her sample were restricted by their domestic commitments.

During the fieldwork I pursued the ideas of providing continuity of care with the midwives who worked in Valley Maternity Hospital. Some of the midwives made comments that were very similar to those reported by Robinson *et al.* as shown in Field note 7.1.

FN 7.1

'Continuity of care is a good idea really, it would be really nice to look after the same woman throughout her pregnancy, labour and after, but it's not really practical.'

'It's not so bad staying on late in the evening, the children are in bed, but well, I don't really like it. I hate going home late at night.'

'I can't stay on in the day. I've got to get home to the kids. Sometimes my husband is on the evening shift, so they are with my mother. Sometimes he wants to go out.'

'I think it would be more satisfying to look after one mother. Perhaps I would learn more and gain more confidence. I will probably be more flexible when my children are older.'

This study began with the premise that the ideal of total continuity was probably unrealistic and unworkable for the majority of midwives and until such times as greater continuity could be achieved through better organised teams, it was worth looking in more detail at traditional methods of care with a view to suggesting improvements.

□ Working shifts

At the Valley Maternity Hospital the twenty four hour cycle was divided into three shifts – 7.00 a.m.–2.30 p.m., 2.00 p.m.–9.30 p.m. and 9.00 p.m.–7.30 a.m. There was a thirty-minute overlap between each shift when the handover took place.

Each of the handover periods, 7.00 a.m., 2.00 p.m. and 9.00 p.m. were observed at least five or six times. I decided to note carefully how the handover was given, where it was given, what was said to whom and their replies, who was excluded from and included in the conversation, and finally I tried to observe what else was happening at the same time. This observation produced a wealth of data and was analysed by devising a typology of handovers.

■ A typology of handovers

It appeared that at the Valley Maternity Hospital there were five quite distinct types of handover. These were classified as:

1. The preamble;
2. The shopping list or just a quickie!
3. Rhythm and jargon;
4. Just the facts;
5. Tender loving care.

Each type is illustrated with data from the field notes.

□ The preamble

The Sister-in-charge would give the Sister who was coming on duty an overview of all the day's work. She would often tell her of all her shift's cases even though they were erased from the board and represented work that was completed. The women had delivered and had been transferred to the post-natal ward. If the shift had dealt with women they considered to be particularly interesting – and that usually meant abnormal – then the Sister-in-charge would describe the cases, the management and outcome in more graphic detail, e.g. 'We had a "brow" this morning. You ought to have seen the baby's head.' or 'We had two emergency sections in the night. One after the other.'

Sometimes the Sister would refer to other women who were 'inpatients' in the maternity unit. These might be potentially abnormal cases. Sometimes, but not always, the details of the case would be written on the board under the section 'messages'. For example, Gravida 8, would be written on the board and the Sister would refer to this woman as 'the Gravida 8 on Ward X is niggling'. Although the details were not always included on the notice-board, most staff would have heard through the grapevine about these women.

The Sister would say 'the twins have delivered'. She would not refer to the woman by name, but the staff coming on duty would clearly be aware of the case and reply 'Oh, good, what did she have?' – a question which referred to the sex of the babies recently born.

It was clear that this period served two distinct purposes: it provided the staff with a general update, and gave information of the 'cases' dealt with and pending.

It was also important for each shift to inform the next shift of the details of the workload that they had coped with. The night shift who were going off duty at 7.00 a.m. were anxious to let the day staff arriving on duty, know how hard they had worked during their shift, e.g. 'It was really hectic last night. One after another, we were up to our eyes.' Sometimes they would apologise that the labour ward was in a mess and would justify this by describing in detail all the cases that they had dealt with during the night.

All the oncoming shifts were suitably sympathetic and made consoling comments, e.g. 'You look exhausted. Don't worry about the mess, we will clear it up.' or 'Don't stay on now, it's late. Off you go, have a good rest.'

Each shift would go to some lengths to explain the extent and the nature of their workload. This appeared to prompt the sympathy of the next shift. This was a very important aspect of the handover. It was an opportunity to be praised and thanked and to receive an acknowledgment of work well done. It seemed that each shift appreciated the comments made by the next shift. It was a time for praise and support and illustrated the very good relationship and close camaraderie that existed between members of the labour ward staff.

□ **The shopping list or just a quickie!**

In this type of handover, a brief summary of the information would be passed from one Sister to another. This usually happened in the corridor, often whilst the Sister who was coming on duty removed her coat. When it was very busy and the next shift's help and expertise were immediately required, this would be the handover in total. The midwife would direct the staff and they would go immediately to the delivery rooms. More commonly, however, this type of handover was an introduction to the handover proper and it would follow the lines shown in Field note 7.2.

FN 7.2 _____

'I'll just give you a quickie report, okay.'

'We've got four in labour, two primips both okay, both had Pethidine. Two multips are cracking on. They won't be any bother.'

'There are two nigglers on the wards, not doing much. There is a niggler over there (pointing to the niggling room), Gravida 2, she's got backache, that's all.'

'Hi, how are you? We've got a breech "fully".'

'Four in labour, none of them doing much, all primips. I expect you will be going walkies later.'

'We've got two. Gravida 4 won't be long, Gravida 2 just got going.'

Nigglers are referred to in more detail in Chapter 6. 'Going walkies' was an interesting phrase as it was a euphemism for delivery by Caesarian section. The operating theatre was situated in the main hospital and women who were to be delivered in this way, would be transferred by trolley, along corridors, to the operating theatre. They would be accompanied by the midwife. The staff, I noted, would be reluctant to discuss this option with the woman. They would talk in whispers and refer to the event as 'going walkies'.

Other comments require further explanation. 'Cracking on' meant that the women referred to were making rapid progress in labour and would be delivering within a short space of time. It was interesting to note how women were classified according to how much work was likely to be involved in completing the case, e.g. 'won't be any bother' and 'should be okay'.

'Fully', it will be recalled, is an abbreviation of the expression 'the cervix is fully dilated'. This signifies the beginning of the second stage of labour. A 'breech fully' is a potentially dangerous birth. The baby, presenting buttocks first, was about to be born. It was important that the midwife arriving on duty was told quickly the details of the cases. It was also noted that only scant attention was paid at this time to any details about the woman as a person, her family, her needs, aspirations or expectations.

There were good organisational reasons for dealing with women as work or cases to be dealt with. As on a factory floor, components arrive, are dealt with according to pre-determined priorities and are moved on to the next phase. So midwifery and childbirth, it could be argued, are not dissimilar to other worlds of work. This aspect is enlarged upon in Chapter 1 and Chapter 8.

On two occasions I noted a slight variation on the 'shopping list' or 'just a quickie' handover. The large window in the office overlooked the main hospital car park. At 2.00 p.m. on a fine day, I noticed the Sister-in-charge looking out of the window. Suddenly, she waved enthusiastically, and shouted. She had seen two midwives crossing the road from the car park and approaching the building. As they did, she waved and shouted 'Hi, you two, there is only one in labour.'

On the other occasion, alerted by now to this interesting variation, I watched the staff approach the unit. They shouted up at the window 'Are you busy?' The Sister who had been waiting in the window replied 'Yes. it's frantic, we are waiting for you two "to go walkies" '.

I noted that the two midwives then took a short cut and appeared at the fire-escape door. They had no other details or any other form of handover. The Sister who had shouted to the midwives laughed heartily as she closed the window. She said 'I don't know what anyone would think if they had heard all that.'

I was sure it was highly probable that many people walking to the car park had witnessed the handover.

This event was treated as a joke shared by most of the staff. The morning shift gathered around the door as the two midwives coming on duty emerged from the fire escape. The event was only observed at the 2.00 p.m. handover. I surmised it was too cold or dark to open windows at 7.00 a.m. and 9.00 p.m., in the middle of winter.

☐ **Rhythm and jargon**

This type of handover usually involved a student midwife. When a student had been looking after a woman in labour she would be encouraged to give a more detailed handover than 'just a quickie'. This handover would take place in the office and usually followed a similar pattern. The student, often looking a little embarrassed, would pick up the notes and begin. Her voice would take on a rhythmical quality as she almost chanted her speech. She would speak in abbreviations, e.g. 'Obs', which referred to observations taken and recorded. 'EDD' would be said as it was written, 'EDD' and not 'estimated date of delivery'. The date would be said as 'twenty-six, first, eighty-nine'. The question marks would be said as 'query query'. 'Rh' would be said as 'Rh' not 'rhesus'.

The handover would be brief, reasonably factual, and give the student the opportunity to manipulate the labour ward in house jargon. It was also noted that the more senior the student midwife, the greater would be her use of the jargon.

Field note 7.3 recalls the details of two such handovers.

The purpose of this ritual was unclear. The students explained that the prospect of the handover filled them with dread during the first days on the labour ward. One student explained to me that she would always try to be 'unavoidably delayed', so as to avoid having to give this performance. On one occasion, it was nearing report time when I was assisting a student

---

FN 7.3

'Well, this is Mrs Smith. Um. She is a Gravida 3, para 2, EDD 26.1.89. Pregnancy normal. Rh. positive. Came in in labour. Had a show. Had a VE. She is 6 centimetres. Had Pethidine. Obs okay.'

and from the more senior student midwife:

'This is a Gravida 5, para 2, one SB. Has been in with IUGR. Had low FMs. In for ECTG and ?? induction. No PE, EDD 3.3.89. Seems SFD. I expect they will get her going later.'

---

with a woman who was labouring on her knees on the floor of the delivery suite. The woman said she wanted to sit in the chair. I offered to help her so that the student could give her handover. She explained, she would much rather I went to the office and gave her apologies for being unavoidably delayed. This I did. Another student told me that the 'doing-a-turn handover', as she explained it, improved with seniority. As she became more experienced she felt less intimidated by having to 'perform for the Sisters'.

All the students to whom I spoke felt there was little educational value in the exercise. Another explained it as yet another example of 'do what I say and not what I do'. She explained that she felt it was ridiculous to give a report in that detail when no one could take in the detail. She said 'After all, when we qualify, we will do it like they do, won't we?'

Is this yet another example of the theory practice gap? Was there a good reason for requiring a handover to include all that detail? I could not see one and felt that a handover which demonstrated the students' ability to analyse and reflect on aspects of care would have been a more useful exercise but the ability to demonstrate the use of jargon served another purpose.

In order to become part of any organisation or system it is necessary to know and demonstrate aspects of the cultural norms of the organisation. When students could give a report in the specified manner, they were no longer outsiders, but part of the team.

They had 'gone native', were more comfortable and could begin to learn. One student told me that after one impressive performance, a Sister had patted her on the back and said 'well done'. The student explained that she felt like 'part of the in-crowd' and that it was worth going through the performance to achieve that status.

□ **Just the facts**

This was the most commonly observed type of handover. It was observed very frequently. It was usually preceded by the 'preamble' previously described and the 'shopping list' or 'just a quickie' type of handover, i.e.

the new midwife would at this stage be aware of the most general details of the case, e.g. 'Gravida 2, getting on'. In this type of handover the cervix was never reported to be more than 7 centimetres dilated (10 centimetres is full dilated and signifies the onset of the second stage).

In the labour ward office the midwife coming on duty would be given a report about the woman she was about to look after. This report would include more detail than the brief summary she would have had whilst she removed her coat. Field note 7.4 illustrates this type of handover.

FN 7.4

'Right. Mrs A. is a Gravida 2; she came in this morning in labour. We did a VE and she is 5 centimetres. She had Pethidine 100 mg at 12 noon and is coping well.'

This handover did not include the amount of detail relating to the woman's obstetric history that the student midwife was expected to state. It was brief, to the point and included the briefest of details.

After the handover, the midwife would leave the office and go to the delivery room. Field note 7.5 illustrates what often happened next:

FN 7.5

Sister 1, the midwife who has been looking after Mrs A. is off duty at 2.30 p.m. The midwife who has just come on duty, Sister 2, walks into the delivery room accompanied by a student midwife who has also just come on duty. They do not 'knock and wait' as the sign asks.

Mrs A. is lying on the bed. She is in established labour. I have just heard, in the report handover, that her cervix is now 5 centimetres dilated. Her contractions are frequent and strong. The student picks up and reads the partogram. She does not speak to Mrs A. or her partner. Sister 1. who is going off duty, asks me when I am going. I tell her I will be staying a little longer today. She leaves the room and does not speak to Mrs A. 'Do you think I'll get this case?' the student asks Sister 2. 'Oh, I expect so' she replies. 'She should deliver by 9.00 p.m. How many more cases do you need?' 'Twelve or thirteen' replies the student.

Sister 2 glances at the partogram and then leaves the room. The student then speaks to the woman for the first time. 'I'm just going to take your blood pressure.'

It would appear that the Sister believed (and the student followed her example) that there was no need to attempt to establish a rapport with the woman at this comparatively early stage of labour. On this occasion, there was no attempt to talk to Mrs A. and though I waited for almost an hour, the student, with the midwife popping in and out, merely carried out the tasks of checking blood pressure, listening and recording the fetal heart rate, etc. Later, I asked the student about Mrs A. I wanted to know why she did not speak to the woman. The student said she had recently been in trouble with Sister 2 because she had failed to complete the partogram. I recorded her answer and it is shown in Field note 7.6.

FN 7.6

'I was worried about getting the job done. Mrs A. seemed quite drowsy and was "coping well". She was not distressed. I didn't want to disturb her and didn't want to get into trouble with Sister 2. There are so many things to remember to do – it's more than just the obs. Two in one. I suppose it's really hard sometimes.'

I then asked her if I had inhibited her in some way and prevented her from talking to the woman. She was sure I had not and that her priority was to complete the partogram.

During other observations following the standard 'just the facts' handover it was noted that often the midwife would have responsibility for more than one woman. Sometimes a student midwife or even a student nurse would be left with the woman with little guidance on how to cope. It seemed clear that the senior midwives (Sisters usually) did not get too involved with the care of women at this stage of labour. Their involvement seemed to be more of a supervisory nature.

The final handover in this typology is called 'Tender Loving Care'.

□ Tender loving care

This type of handover was, it seemed, reserved for those women who had sufficiently progressed in labour to warrant such attention. The cervix was always reported to be more than 7 centimetres dilated. An initial brief handover ('Just a quickie' or 'the shopping list') would have taken place as usual in the labour ward office. If, during this report the staff indicated that a woman in labour had progressed to 7 centimetres or more, an additional and much more detailed handover would subsequently take place. This fifth type of handover always took place in the delivery room at the woman's bedside. The exchange of information would be much more detailed. The first midwife would introduce the second midwife coming on duty to the woman in labour and often to her partner. Often they would use Christian names. This is the first time that the woman in labour was included in the handover. The handover would include social chitchat with the woman and less attention would be paid to the technicalities of the progress of labour. The second midwife would often introduce herself by name and explain that she had just arrived on duty and would tell the woman what time she would be going home. They would all – i.e. the midwife leaving, the midwife arriving, the woman and her partner – chat together. The midwife who was coming on duty would explain to the woman and her partner that she would be responsible for the care of the family until after the baby was born. There would often be discussion about weather, the news, the woman's other children and who was caring for them. The midwife would often ask the partner if he had had a drink or something to eat. The midwife and the woman would often discuss names for the baby and even aspects of how the woman wanted the birth to be conducted. There were no formal birth plans but frequently in this handover at a relatively late stage of labour there would be discussion about pain relief, episiotomy, use of syntometrine and even if the mother would prefer the baby delivered directly into her arms or washed and dried first. The student would join in the conversation often explaining some details of her training to the family, as she completed the observations. The atmosphere seemed positive and supportive. The midwife would stay with the woman. I did not observe any written evidence of this positive communication and it was always only when the cervix was dilated to over 7 centimetres, that I was able to witness this kind of handover.

■ Home time

I tried to record the parting words of the midwife who was going off duty and Field notes 7.7 give a flavour of the atmosphere and warmth of these exchanges and demonstrate the hold on control. The midwife going off duty would explain her departure and leave with a parting comment such as those listed.

FN 7.7

'Well love, I thought I would have had you today, but it looks as if you are going to be the night shift's. Be good, and do what they tell you.'

'Look kid, I've done my whack now. This is Sister 3, do what she says and you will be all right.'

'Listen Mary, I'm off now. Sister 4 will take care of you. I'll see you tomorrow when the baby is in the cot.'

'It's been a long day, Susi, but everything is going well now. Sister 5 is a great midwife and you will be fine with her.'

'What a night. You have kept us going, I'm sorry I can't stay. Midwife 6 will take good care of you now. Don't worry. It's all going fine.'

'Good-bye Mrs M. Hope all goes well. Sister 8 is looking after you know. Take care, I'll see you without the bump.'

This fifth type of handover was most interesting. The examples taken from the field notes illustrate how the midwives view this stage of labour. The second stage of labour, the delivery, and the period immediately preceding it, that is, when the cervix is between 7 and 10 centimetres dilated, represents the focus of the delivery suite work. It was the high point of the midwife's work and the event with which many other aspects of the labour ward were closely related.

It seemed that on a busy labour ward, work did not become real work, important work, requiring personal intervention and sole contact with the woman, until labour was well-advanced and birth likely to occur within a short time.

The midwife involved in this stage was entitled to wear the 'badge of blood' as described in Chapter 5, be rewarded with tea as described in Chapter 6 and even be granted temporary immunity from further work. Careful individual attention of women in labour was only granted when the work became real.

This aspect of the study indicated quite clearly that at the Valley Maternity Hospital, the quality of the handover, its length and location were directly related to the dilation of the cervix.

If care cannot be reorganised to provide the continuity of care that women are asking for, then midwives could be advised to reconsider the way in which handovers take place during labour. There is no doubt that the effects of discontinuity cannot be more acute than when a woman is in well-established labour.

■ Shifts, stresses and strains

Towards the end of the fieldwork stage of the study I decided to conduct some more in-depth interviews with the some of the midwives. These interviews aimed to confirm some of the emerging theories particularly in relation to the handover and to discover more of the culture of Valley Maternity Hospital midwifery.

It was around midday late in March when I arrived on the unit, there was no one in labour and the atmosphere seemed relaxed. The office was more organised then usual and the notice-board was wiped clean. There had not been any births that morning and this had given the staff the opportunity to 'get straight'. The routine administrative tasks of ordering the pharmacy, etc., had been completed and the only 'niggler' had been transferred to the antenatal ward. Tea was being made and when I arrived I was greeted warmly and offered a drink. I explained that I was nearing the end of the fieldwork stage of the study but now wanted to discuss some aspects in more detail. I had planned to interview Sister 6 alone but as two staff midwives seemed anxious to join in the discussion I proceeded on that basis.

I began by asking Sister 6 what did she liked most about her job. She said that she enjoyed being a midwife most of the time and generally had a high level of job satisfaction. She said that she had worked at Valley for some years and generally 'they' left her alone. I asked who 'they' were and she explained that she meant the medical staff and offered the additional information that the midwifery managers did not cause her much trouble.

She went on to explain that she enjoyed the company of her colleagues and students and liked the discipline and order of her job. She added that she enjoyed her contact with the women. I asked her to explain further what she meant by 'discipline and order'. She said that she felt there was a right way to do things and that was the way things must be done. I asked what she meant by 'things'. She said 'I mean the charts, the labour ward records, the Birth Register' and then she said 'I am happiest when women come in in labour, they get on with it, have a normal baby and get off to the wards. That is when I feel I have done a good job.' She went on to explain how it was good to be in charge and when she managed to avoid what she described as 'unnecessary interference'.

I was keen to explore more of the positive aspects of being a midwife but my informants were anxious to tell me more of the stresses and negative features of being a midwife.

The Sister said that she strongly disliked the pressure of the job which she considered was aggravated by frequent staff shortages. She said that often she went home feeling frustrated by the fact that she had not done the job properly. She said 'You cannot give good care to three women at once, you bob in and out, solve problems and move on'; she felt that it was not right for women to be left alone in labour or to be cared for only by student midwives. She said that she felt students had a 'rough deal' and were not taught properly. She explained that the students were often used as pairs of hands and 'learnt on the job'. She then went to express her frustration with what she described as 'being constrained by the system'. I recorded her comments and they are in Field note 7.8.

FN 7.8

'I dislike the Consultants, one day they trust me and say they agree with my decisions and another day they come in and give me a list of instructions like a monkey in a cage. It's not as if they don't know me but they don't always trust me. If we let them [the consultants] decide on everything they soon will not need midwives except perhaps at night – they will not get out of bed for normal labour. Anyone can follow rules and protocols but what is the point of training and passing exams when the system asks you not to think?'

I listened carefully and only intervened to seek clarification or more information. Sister went on to explain that she felt it was important for midwives to keep their independent role; in her opinion they should act responsibly and on their own initiative. She took the opportunity to explain to the two staff midwives that they were accountable for their practice regardless of whose name was stamped on the woman's note. It was clearly sometimes frustrating to be a midwife at the Valley Maternity Hospital. The midwives' oft-repeated phrase and belief of being 'a practitioner in their own right' was frequently frustrated by a system that imposed rules and constraints on practice. The Sisters clearly felt that they had the ability and experience to break free and to use their initiative. It seemed that they often found ways around the system and exerted their own controls.

I then decided to explore further the issue of working shifts and the events that surrounded the handover.

I spoke to the staff midwives to try to obtain their views on the handover and on working late, past their normal finishing time. Field note 7.9 is a transcript of an interview with a staff midwife. She describes the handover and gives her opinion on aspects of continuity of care. I wanted to know how this staff midwife would deal with the problem of handing over the care of a woman before the care was completed, particularly if she had established a special relationship with the women involved.

This interview was conducted in the labour ward office one evening in January. The staff midwife who was on duty talked to me whilst she made some sandwiches and drank her tea. She said she was keen to talk to me and did not mind the tape-recorder.

In this interview the staff midwife explained the details of the handover and confirmed the observational data. A handover would only take place in the delivery room if the woman was feeling 'pushy'. (In the second stage of labour the woman will experience expulsive contractions, or if the cervix is dilated by more than 7 centimetres.) She paid scant attention to the particular wishes of the woman in labour, explaining that if she did get an 'awkward one' – that is someone who wanted something different (obviously a deviant!) she would merely tell the Sister-in-charge and record the fact.

She went on to explain her feelings about staying on duty past her normal finishing time in order to give the woman in labour the benefit of her continuous care. She explained that her criterion was usually whether she liked the woman or not. She explained that she was usually tired but may, if she felt she was getting on well with the woman, stay on duty.

This was probably a quite reasonable response. It would be expected that if the midwife was enjoying the experience and did not have any demanding domestic circumstances, she would be more likely to remain on duty and complete the care of the woman.

The next interview, with the senior Sister-in-charge of the labour ward, considers further the aspect of staying on duty after a shift has ended. This interview was tape-recorded and then transcribed, as in Field note 7.10.

FN 7.9

(Researcher = *R*; Midwife = *M*)

R: Your shift finishes at 9.30 p.m. tonight?

M: Yes, that's right, we usually do two or three lates and two earlies.

R: If you are looking after someone in labour would you hand the care over to another midwife at 9 p.m.?

M: Yes, I'm usually keen to go by then.

R: Where do you normally give the handover?

M: Well, in here, everything happens in the office. Well, but if she is well on in labour or say a multip – you know – it just depends. Sometimes in the office, sometimes in the labour ward.

R: Can you explain what you mean by 'well on'?

M: Well, you know – feeling 'pushy'!

R: So if she was feeling 'pushy' you would hand over in the labour ward?

M: Well, yes. Unless there was someone else around to stay with her.

R: Can you give me an example?

M: Well, her husband, but I would prefer a nursing auxiliary, you know someone who would come and get me if it was urgent.

R: You also said that if she was a 'multip' you might not give the report in the office.

M: No, well . . . I think I would only give a report in there [the delivery room] if she was going to just push it out! [she laughs] Really if I thought a multip was more than 7 centimetres I would probably hand over quickly in the office and again in the labour ward.

R: Thank you. Can you tell me more about the handover? Is there anything special or anything in particular that you would need to tell the next midwife?

M: Well, nothing really, just to say when she came in – oh, what her name is; primip or multip; any complications. Um, well, basically haemoglobin, blood group, rubella, what she came in with – and, well – her progress.

R: What would you do if you were looking after someone in labour who had asked for something special, e.g. when the cord was to be cut, or giving or not wanting a particular drug to be administered?

M: Oh, no one wants anything special here, you get some awkward ones, but you just tell the Sister-in-charge and write it in the notes.

R: What would you do if the woman you were looking after reached the second stage of labour at 9.00 p.m?

M: Well, now you have put me on the spot. Put it this way, if you like her you stay on, you know. Well, if you don't like her, or don't get on with her, well you don't. Sometimes you get a woman who you are keen to leave behind, you know, eager to pass her on. Especially if its late and you are on early the next day. Sister stayed on once all day 7.00 a.m. to 9.30 p.m. – she was looking after a doctor's wife. She was shattered and no one thanked her for it.

R: Thank you very much, that has been really helpful.

FN 7.10

(Researcher = *R*; Sister = *S*)

R: 'Sister, when you are in charge of the labour ward and the time of a shift change approaches, how do you feel about the midwives staying on duty past their normal finishing time, in order to stay with the woman they know?

S: Oh, I think it's fine, as long as they are happy to do it, I don't really mind.

R: Do you arrange for them to take time off in lieu or are they paid overtime?

S: Oh, no they never get paid. [Pause]

R: So, if a midwife stays on duty in order to give continuity of care, she does not get paid for it.

S: Yes that's right, this place only keeps going on unpaid overtime.

R: Do you keep a written record of time that is worked in excess of the usual 37.5 hour week?

S: Yes, then if it ever gets quiet, we try to give them the time back . . . [pause] but really the system does not cope; there is a lot of unpaid overtime. It is rare that it is quiet. When it is, we need to catch up on routine work – you know, cleaning, ordering stock, that sort of thing. I think I am owed weeks, not days or hours. The other Sisters as well. It's shameful really.

R: Are the staff midwives in the same position?

S: Yes, some are, but not as much as me. You see I go to meetings and things. I go in my own time.

R: So you feel that all midwives do a lot of unpaid overtime.

S: Yes, but some weeks it's not so busy.

R: Do you think that unpaid overtime is a good or bad thing?

S: Well, it's bad really; they would never pay anyway, they just rely on our dedication I suppose. You know, 'Angels of Mercy' and that sort of stuff.

R: Yes. What would you be most likely to do if the women you were looking after reached the second stage of labour at 9.00 p.m.?

S: Well, I would probably stay – well, it depends really. If she was a primip, maybe not. If she was a multip – well, may be . . . um . . . Actually the 9.00p.m. change is more of a problem. We usually work a late shift, ie 2.30–9.30p.m. followed by an early the next day, that is 7.00a.m.–2.30p.m. – it's really hard to stay on, especially if you are on early the next day. If you deliver at 9.30p.m. it's going to take until at least 10.30p.m. to finish the notes. Lots of them don't like going home that late, even if they drive. You get in late, you are all wound up and then you can't sleep and then you feel a wreck the next day . . . well, really you are more likely to stay on and complete a case at 2.30p.m. than at 9.30p.m.

R: Thank you, that is helpful. Are the night staff likely to stay on in the morning if, say, a delivery is imminent at 7.00a.m.?

S: Well, again I suppose if they were multips they would stay but – well, a lot of these girls have small children, they have to get home and take them to school, let their husbands go to work, give him the car! You know, that's why they work nights.

R: So it would seem that the best chance of a woman having the same midwife throughout labour would be to come in early in the morning and preferably deliver within the time-span of one shift or around 2.00p.m?

S: [Laughing] Yes, that's right.

R: I'm also very interested in the handover at a shift change. Where does the handover take place?

S: Well, usually here in the office. I don't think most people mind a different midwife. You see it's so busy we have women queuing up for labour ward, the nigglers are waiting for a space. I tell the next shift so they know what to expect. As long as someone is around they don't seem to mind.

R: Thank you.

The interview indicates that a woman in labour is more likely to obtain the care of one midwife throughout her labour if she arrives early in the morning and delivers by early afternoon.

Roth (1963) explains that patients in hospital obtain most of their information from other patients. Women who are admitted in labour have no other contact with hospital in-patients. They are moved from the admission room to the delivery suite and unless they find themselves in the 'niggling room', they are denied the opportunity to learn the rules of the organisation. They are forced to rely directly on the midwife for information to orientate themselves to the environment. It is another blow when they find that the midwife with whom they formed a relationship goes off duty and is replaced by yet another stranger.

From the current literature it seems that the consumers are demanding continuity of care and are rejecting 'a different face each time' in the antenatal clinic and during labour. They appear to want the midwifery profession to show an increase in individual responsibility and some personal commitment to women in labour.

Yet, as Zerubavel (1979) comments 'It is one of the major organisational imperatives of bureaucratic complexes such as the hospital, to minimise the total indispensability and irreplaceability of a particular physician, or nurse as much as possible.'

It could be argued that running a system on unpaid overtime whilst relying on the goodwill of midwives is an example of the way a hospital bureaucracy works. It attempts to minimise the indispensability and irreplaceability of the midwives, by organising a system of shifts that does not allow for continuity of care.

As the field notes illustrate, it is not practical to stay late on duty, after 9.00p.m. to care for a woman in labour until her child is born when the same midwife is expected back on duty at 7.00a.m. the next morning, nor to stay on at 7.30a.m. after working on an eleven-hour shift. The shift system that removes one midwife and replaces her with another after seven-and-a-half hours may be said to encourage her to feel both replaceable and dispensable.

Detailed analysis of the shift handover illustrates certain inadequacies in the way the information was exchanged at the Valley Maternity Hospital. Women described as 'nigglers' were not kept informed and did not know who was responsible for their care. Women in labour who had not progressed beyond the stage where their cervix was dilated to 7 centimetres were not afforded the benefit of a handover which would assist both woman and midwife in understanding each other and establishing some sort of relationship. The time allocated to the handover could have been used much more effectively to minimise the adverse effects of the fragmented care currently available.

■ The agony of advocacy

Another theme emerged during conversations with the midwives which is worth recording. On one occasion a group of staff midwives had gathered in the office, it was around 8p.m. and their shift was nearly over. The labour ward was quiet and most of the cleaning and checking of equipment was complete.

The conversation focused on the phrase 'a practitioner in their own right'. This is a much-quoted phrase and one where the real meaning is often left vague. They explained that they felt the power of being independent autonomous practitioners the most when they were left alone and undisturbed by medical interventions. Like the midwives on night duty they enjoyed the freedom to practice, to assess, to plan, implement and evaluate care; they said that they felt this most when they were involved in the management of normal birth.

However, freedom, power and control had another dimension. This I have called the agony of advocacy. When the midwives were involved in the care of women in labour and in hospital, some felt that they knew very clearly that they had the power to influence the quality of the childbirth experience. The power of practice and the power over practice was in some ways frightening. The emotional strength that was required to act as a woman's advocate was described as considerable. Some of the midwives explained that during the birth experience they felt that they became part of that woman's experience. They said that on those occasions they were totally 'with woman'. They described how working alongside her was physically and mentally draining. If the situation deviated from normal and an intervention was planned, or a routine procedure was due, e.g. an 'unnecessary' vaginal examination, then they had to step outside their role of 'midwife-with woman' and become an 'advocate'. The words of one midwife tape-recorded and transcribed in Field note 7.11 describes this well.

FN 7.11

'You develop a very close relationship with a woman during her labour, you are with her, sweating with her, alongside her, supporting, caring, rubbing her back, listening, watching, feeling. You become part of that experience. As the midwife you have the power to decide the quality, it can be good, bad or just okay. It's in your hands. Sometimes you have to step outside the intensity of the relationship, you have to be an advocate. Sometimes you are challenged by the medical staff, the SHOs are easy but the Registrars are difficult and authoritarian.When you challenge a Registrar you step outside your position of power and control. Outside it is difficult, very difficult. It's challenging and painful. It is easier to comply. It's much easier just to do the routines or rupture the membranes, so you ease back, you retreat into a world where you can be in control. Where you feel that you can be a "practitioner in your own right". It is not always easy and often the women don't get the best possible care. The doctors are more powerful than any woman or midwife. Female doctors can sometimes be worse than male. It is as if they have something more to prove. Anyway the end result is often that the women's wants, needs and even rights are swallowed up in procedures and routines. Even the strongest, most assertive and articulate midwives can crumple under that sort of strain. Who wins? Certainly not women.'

Another midwife also explained that the power of the obstetricians was always too great. She said:

> We are always threatened with litigation. They say if anything goes wrong the Doctors carry the can. The UKCC say we are [accountable] so I'm not sure. When I come out of being 'with woman' and act as her advocate it is much more uncomfortable for me. I would rather just work for a quiet life.

This section presents an interesting view of the topic of autonomy and accountability. The legal position of midwives was seen as unclear and although they felt the power of practice, it seemed that they were unable or unwilling to use that power as advocates for women, they retreated from the agony of advocacy preferring to follow orders rather than challenge the power of the medical staff.

■ Working at night

The fieldwork stage of this ethnographic study also included observation of life on night duty at Valley Maternity Hospital. As previously recorded, observation in the field began with some questions. I was interested to know why some midwives worked a permanent night shift and also if there were any significant features of night duty.

The shift began at 9p.m. and a period of thirty minutes was allowed for the handover to take place. I arrived at 8.45p.m. and gave my usual introduction to new faces.

During the first night of observation two midwives were allocated to the labour ward; there was also a student midwife. The Sister who was on night duty said that they were 'well staffed for a change'. She explained that she could call on the help of nursing auxiliaries, if required, but that most of the staff began their shift on the wards. Later, when most of the work was completed and the mothers and babies were settled, most of the staff would return to the labour ward, leaving only one or two staff midwives or nursing auxiliaries on the wards. The night staff were also responsible for all other maternity 'in-patients', those awaiting their babies and those delivered.

There were considerably fewer medical staff around at night, no administrators, senior managers, clerks, visitors, partners and, most notably, no meals to be given out to the women on the wards. The night staff allocated to the labour ward were responsible for the care of women in labour and were not expected to be involved in ordering stores, drugs and equipment. They were, however, responsible for ensuring they had sufficient stocks, e.g. drugs, intravenous fluids, etc., and that their equipment was in good order. The midwives were observed carefully checking resuscitation equipment. The night routines were interesting in that they illustrated how the staff coped with heat, the length of the shift and the fact that medical assistance, if required, was not as immediately available as it was during the day.

On my first visit there were two women in labour and the handover followed the style previously described. The 'preamble' was followed by 'just the facts' and, because in this case a Mrs J. was well-advanced in labour, a further 'tender loving care' type of handover followed. This took place in the delivery room. It was a very warm and very small room and appeared crowded with the midwives and Mrs J.'s partner. Mrs J. was well-advanced in labour, her cervix being some 8 centimetres dilated. Her care was handed from day-shift midwife to night-shift midwife in her presence. It was obvious that a warm relationship existed between the day midwife, the woman and her partner. The midwife's parting shot was: 'Cheerio J . . . I'm sure everything will be okay. I'll see you tomorrow. Do what the midwife says and you will be okay. Has your old man got enough fags?' She left smiling and laughing to J's husband.

Mr J. was a tall heavily built man who looked uncomfortable and ill-at-ease in the corner of the room. He was wearing jeans and a T-shirt. When the night midwives came into the room, he quickly stood up and moved towards the door. In his hand was a packet of cigarettes. He held it up to the midwife and gestured that he wanted to leave to have a smoke. He waited by the door until the night midwife said 'Go on, off you go.' It appeared that he needed her permission to leave the room. Mrs J. was resting between her strong contractions, her eyes were closed. The night Sister appeared to be in charge and listened carefully to the handover.

Mrs J. occasionally opened her eyes and acknowledged the fact that the night Sister was taking over her care. At one point she said 'Where is Joe?', the night midwife said 'I've told him he is allowed a quick smoke.' The right of exit was controlled by the Sister.

Between 9p.m. and 11p.m. I felt that I observed very little difference between day and night shifts. All the lights were on in the delivery suite and the radio continued to turn out popular music. After 11p.m., however, it seemed to be a different world. The medical staff were much less in evidence. A young SHO drifted in, yawned and looked at the blackboard, 'Much business?' he asked. I replied that I would get the Sister if it would help. He yawned again and said 'No, it's okay' and he left the unit. I am sure he had no idea who I was but I was in the backstage area of the office and not challenged. This action, even though it was early in the night, was in marked contrast to the behaviour of medical staff that I had observed during the day.

At this time there was a greater chance of the chief (the consultant) appearing so the junior doctors would spend more time in checking on the details of all women in labour. As the SHO left, he said 'They will bleep if they need me.' During the day I had observed that he would have been more likely to have investigated the workload more thoroughly. He wandered off and did not go into any of the delivery rooms. He seemed very tired.

The night Sister would usually allocate herself to the delivery suite, whilst another Sister would oversee the care on the wards. On one occasion there was only one Sister on the unit and it was her job both to supervise the labour ward and oversee the care on both the wards. The staff midwives and the student took a case each. (A case being one woman in labour.) There were two women in labour at that time. The case of Mrs J., who was most advanced in labour was allocated to the student midwife so that 'She could get her cases.' The Sister said to the staff midwife 'Can you keep an eye on the student till I get back?' The staff midwife was allocated to the care of the second woman in labour, Mrs A., who, though making slow progress in labour, was not considered to be a complicated case.

Almost as soon as Sister disappeared, the staff midwife returned to the office to put the kettle on. This was not, I discovered, because Sister was not there, but as explained by the staff midwife: 'God, it's hot in there. I'm dying of thirst. Do you want a cuppa?' I thanked her but declined on this occasion. I was about to ask if it was usual to stop at this time for tea, when she said 'We usually have a drink now, especially if its quiet – you see it might be hectic later.' I reflected that I considered the unit to be quite busy at that time and that the student who was involved in the care of Mrs J. might need supervision and some support. However, the staff midwife told me, 'We drink lots of tea on nights, you can get so dehydrated in the heat on such a long shift.' I agreed and sympathised with the organisation of shifts that had resulted in an eleven-hour night shift. By 11p.m., the atmosphere of the unit had changed considerably. The lights were extinguished in the corridors and main rooms. In the delivery rooms, only small lights were on above the beds. The radio was switched off. It was quiet and apart from the staff midwife and student, there was no one around. There were no domestics on night duty. There was no routine cleaning and when the telephone rang it seemed much louder than when it rang during the day. The atmosphere was generally more tranquil and relaxed.

Night duty, it seemed, provided the midwife with a greater opportunity to act as an independent practitioner and to come closer to a degree of professional autonomy. She was still restricted by the policies dictated by the consultants but the lack of the physical presence of medical staff, unless summoned, gave her greater scope. It seemed very clear that at night, the labour ward belonged to the midwives, it was their world and their area of authority and power.

Many of the midwives, whom I interviewed, who work permanently on the night shift, did so because of limited interference by medical staff. They described the greater freedom and the support that they had for each other. They commented on how much they liked being able to make decisions and be responsible for the care of a woman without medical intervention. It was their decision when to call in medical aid and when to act on their own initiative, One Sister's explanation is given in Field note 7.12.

FN 7.12

'On day-duty, the medical staff do rounds. They look at the partogram and suggest interventions. For example, if a woman is 4 centimetres and her membranes are still intact, they always write in the notes ARM at the next VE. At night, they don't do rounds, so they don't interfere. Most of us think that an ARM is unnecessary at 4 centimetres. The women cope better if the membranes are left intact until later. We have all seen them go out of control and up the wall with pain after an ARM. So at night its easy, what they don't see or don't know about they don't worry about.'

ARM: Artificial rupture of the amniotic membranes. 4 centimetres refers to the dilatation of the cervix, 4 centimetres is slightly less than 50 per cent dilated.There is some debate in the literature on the value of artificial rupture of the membranes early in labour.

This Sister clearly explained that midwives were the experts in the management of normal labour and appeared to suggest that it was only the nights that she had the opportunity to practise her skill.

Shortly before 11p.m. the student midwife emerged from the delivery room and shouted across the corridor to the staff midwife, who was talking to me. 'We've got a head – she's fully.' The staff midwife who had up until this time been either in the ward with Mrs A., the second mother in labour, or drinking tea, jumped up quickly. She hurried into the delivery room and started to collect bits of equipment. She did not look at Mrs J. – who was somewhat fraught at this time – the monitor or the student. I noted this and considered that as she was the midwife who would be responsible for the care, I had expected her to make a more detailed examination and/or assessment of the woman.

The midwife, however seemed totally confident and later explained to me that she was relying heavily on her experience and gut feeling. As an experienced midwife she said she had made her assessment earlier and knew that Mrs J. was fine and would deliver her baby quite normally within a few hours. I had observed the expert practitioner described by Benner (1984) in action. The student midwife who had been training for only three months or so was opening the delivery pack and then washing her hands. The midwife asked where Mrs J.'s partner was and the student replied that he had gone for a cigarette. The midwife looked at me and by implication suggested I went to find him. This I did. I had previously asked both Mrs J. and her husband if they objected to my being present for the birth of their baby. They did not mind even though the room was even more crowded.

Both the midwife and the student busied themselves preparing for the birth. The following comments seemed to illustrate some of the difference between day and night duty.

'Oh you've timed that well, Mrs J., you will be all cleaned up and asleep by midnight.'

The midwife then turned to the student and said:

'Mine won't be long . . . perhaps we will have a quiet night after this.'

I observed again that it was not uncommon for two members of staff to conduct a conversation in the woman's presence. Their anxiety to 'get through the work, clean up and sit down', was again obvious. This was work, the process of production was an effective labour and the output was to be the baby. Mrs J. had a straightforward birth and in a very short space of time had been transferred to the post-natal ward. The production cycle was complete.

■ More tea? Enter Mrs Brown

Sister had returned from the wards and popped her head into the room where the midwife was attending to Mrs A. who was still in labour. She said 'Mrs Brown's fully.' I looked up expectantly, wondering how I had missed someone else being in advanced labour. I left the delivery room and looked for this third woman. Both the Sister and staff midwife were laughing heartily at my confusion. They said, 'Don't they say that at . . . (the hospital where I worked). I replied that I did not understand. 'Mrs Brown is fully', they explained, meant the tea was made and 'Mrs Brown had delivered' meant that the tea was poured! I was amused at this and reflected that although I had been familiar with a similar code, it was the difference in name that had confused me.

At the hospital where I had worked it was also the usual practice to make tea at fairly regular intervals. It was not difficult to understand why the midwives would not discuss their 'illegal' breaks in front of the woman and her partner, even though they would often bring the woman's relatives a cup of tea.

Even though I was a midwife and very familiar with the other hospital's labour wards, I was a complete outsider when it came to interpreting the code 'Mrs Brown's fully'. It also amused the staff, that as a fellow midwife, I was unaware of the arrangement. Tea-drinking continued to be a major cultural activity of both day duty and night duty.

Sometime later, Mrs A. gave birth. It was around 1a.m.; I was amazed at how many staff seemed to just appear. In record time Mrs A. was 'washed and warded' – an abbreviation for washing the mother, assisting her into her night-clothes, washing and dressing the baby, feeding the baby and transferring both mother and baby to the post-natal ward. 'Washing and warding' was usually the nursing auxiliary's responsibility. However, I was told that on night duty there was an urgency to return the mother to her bed and so an 'all hands on deck' policy was adopted. The staff midwife, student, Sister, two nursing auxiliaries, were all involved with cleaning both Mrs A. and the equipment. There was a real urgency to complete the process. Whilst it made sense for Mrs A. to be helped to return to the ward in order to sleep and recover, it seemed that scant attention was paid to her psychological needs. Birth is a momentous event and many women report that they are unable to sleep immediately following the birth. The woman and her partner needed a period of time together in peace and quiet to begin to adjust to their new lives. Mr and Mrs A. were treated efficiently, Mrs A. was 'washed and warded'. The staff had been efficient but perhaps they were not effective. The urgency to complete the process had overtaken everything else.

Within an hour the staff had assembled in the office. The chairs were arranged in a circle, tea was made (again!) and the staff sat down; most removed their shoes and began to open packs of sandwiches, etc. Sister arrived and said 'Is anything coming in?' Her colleagues assured her that no one was expected. She was advised to 'grab a snack' while it was 'all quiet on the western front'. They chatted in a relaxed way to me about how night duty was different and that although their sleep patterns were disturbed, this was compensated for by three aspects of working night duty. They explained that:

1. There was less medical intervention and interference, and this allowed them more and better opportunity to act as 'midwives' and not as doctors' 'handmaidens'.
2. The 'all hands on deck' policy was peculiar to night duty. They described this as all helping in a 'case'. They contrasted this with day duty where they said an individual midwife was totally responsible for the care of the women.
3. There was an improved camaraderie, and much better interpersonal relationship existed as compared with the day shift.

It became obvious that the hospital hierarchical system had little meaning on night duty. Although traditionally, nursing auxiliaries perform more menial jobs, e.g. washing beds, trolleys and making tea, at night there did seem to be more of a group effort. Sisters were observed performing tasks that during the day mainly formed part of the nursing auxiliary role. Washing the labour ward floor was noted to be a distinct example.

On another occasion when my fieldwork was during the night duty period I noted another minor difference between the day and night shift. It is noted in Field note 7.13.

FN 7.13

Sister S. looked much smarter than usual today. Her hair was neatly pinned up (it usually hangs freely), she wore make-up and her uniform was obviously pressed and clean. She wore perfume and was carrying a shopping basket. She looked almost as if she was out for a trip, not coming to work. It seemed to be more of a social event than day duty.

In my discussions with the night staff much later in the evening they told me that another aspect of night duty they enjoyed was avoiding the 'early morning rush'. They said that they enjoyed having time to 'wash and dress tidy' and 'put a bit of make-up on'. They said that they felt that the day shift began much too early at 7 a.m.

At around 3 a.m. on another visit, the unit again was quiet after a very busy period. It was Saturday night and I was told that it was customary for the staff on duty either to send out to a local take-away for a meal or else to bring in the components of a supper. One of the midwives told me that whenever they planned to do this the unit would be busy. She referred to this phenomenon as 'Sod's Law'. On the night in question, at 3a.m. all the women had been delivered and transferred to wards in the customary way and the group meal had been eaten.

Assembled in the office were two Sisters, a staff midwife and a student. They were sharing a meal and discussing the evening's events and also their past successes and failures. Conversations frequently began with: 'Do you remember that Mrs . . . a Gravida 2 who . . .?' All present joined in with a chorus of comments on the mother's lack of personal hygiene and how they had to ask her to bath before anyone would attend to her. They also commented that this was unusual and that most women bathe before admission. They also commented on the women who were particularly obese or who had limited intelligence. Another series of comments was reserved for the somewhat unusual admission of women of an ethnic minority group.

On more than one occasion I heard the same joke being made about women who wore saris or silk trousers and how this restricted the midwives' activities. Ethnic minority groups were very rare admissions at Valley Maternity Hospital.

Night duty offered during its quieter periods, greater opportunities for the staff to reminisce about their past success and failures. It appeared that more recent births were discussed first and then as time went on, the conversations dealt with momentous events of the past. I heard on more than one occasion the same story about a particularly traumatic delivery with unsuccessful outcome. Births were recalled and could be classified in the following way. All the staff described the births using the same typology.

(a) *Successful*: in these cases there was no medical intervention and the woman's wishes were satisfied. The midwife would describe her feelings as good, and well-satisfied with the outcome.

(b) *Could have been better*: in these cases there was some medical intervention (not always considered by midwife to be necessary). The woman would have experienced a positive end result, i.e. a live baby and the midwife would comment, 'if only they had followed my advice it would have been okay'. For example: 'Do you remember Mrs K? She was in labour for hours. We kept ringing them and they wouldn't section her.' In the end she had an emergency section for fetal distress.

(c) *Terrible cases*: In these cases there was always maximum medical involvement. The delivery was often traumatic for mother and baby, e.g. a large episiotomy, a very low Apgar score at the time of birth, and always some form of medical intervention that was, in the opinion of the midwife, too little, too late. For example: 'What about Mrs H? That was terrible. Kept her hanging on – only because she was 16 and unmarried. She ends up with a failed forceps and section. Baby Apgar 2. It makes you sick.'

Discussions of this nature were only observed during quiet periods on night duty. The observations recorded in the field notes describe what midwives do but also give a good description of how they describe and define their expertise and competencies to each other. The reminiscences on night duty were particularly useful in this respect. Dingwall (1977) further describes this phenomenon in 'Atrocity Stories and Professional Relationships'.

The midwives working on night duty at Valley Maternity Hospital were vocal and assertive. They would argue vigorously about the rights and wrongs of the management of the birth process. They frequently expressed their frustration with the medical interventionist type of care. They were confident about the management of normal birth and frustrated with the junior medical staff. As one Sister put it 'When I tell them I want them to come I want them now and not after they have argued the toss.'

Night duty was different from day duty in many ways. The working relationship between the midwives and other support staff was much closer. Many chose to work on night duty because in that system this gave them greater freedom and autonomy. Some worked on night duty because it fitted in with their family and because it was better paid than day duty. All the staff explained that the atmosphere of night duty was warmer, closer, less judgemental and more supportive. This is perhaps what happens to teams of midwives when they work closely together.

Chapter 8

Reflections and conclusions

This study began with a scene-setting section which attempted to place the meaning of midwifery as a female professional project within a set of historical and social conditions. After a reading of the ethnographic study of a labour ward culture it is important to draw out some of the themes which have emerged and to examine them in more detail. What, if any, conclusions can be drawn?

Two main themes dominated the backdrop to the research; first, the policy moves and sets of ideas which led to the site of childbirth to be placed in hospital, and second, the strategies which midwifery undertook as an upwardly striving female professional project. These two factors, it has been argued, have been significant in setting and informing the composition of a working culture which daily reinforces and recreates an individual and collective occupational identity. For it is through this culture with its beliefs, attitudes and actions that each generation learns what it 'means' to be a midwife. As Paul Willis (1979) states:

> Culture is not artifice and manners, the preserve of Sunday best, rainy afternoons and concert halls. It is the very material of our daily lives, the bricks and mortar of our most commonplace understandings, feelings and responses.

This is not to suggest that the labour ward culture is a universal one or that individuals do not set up strategies of resistance within organisations but it does represent an attempt to isolate certain characteristics which are inherent in the hospital-based production process.

It would however, be a gross over-simplification to make the equation,

'Site = Culture'

for in so doing, many important elements would be overlooked. In order to avoid this deterministic conclusion a further element needs to be thought through, this being the crucial one of the relationship between a 'professional' occupation and women in a patriarchal culture.

■ Culture and production

Throughout this study, the organisation of hospital birth has been likened to that of the factory production process. This has meant that aspects of the social and cultural relations of production have been incorporated into the day-to-day working experiences of midwives. The shift system, the line-management structure, the emphasis on production targets and the attempts to regularise an unpredictable work-pattern are all familiar components of an industrial setting.

The daily strategies for 'getting through' the work, the interface rivalries, the language and the jokes, presentation of strength and endurance, the ways of 'slowing down' the line, all these are echoed in other recorded experiences of masculinised industrial work (Beynon, 1973; Willis, 1979). Ruth Cavendish (1982) in her description of women working on the assembly line showed that as well as similarities there are some essential differences in a female experience of the production process. Women are workers in this setting of the public world of work and at the same time they occupy another space within the private world of the home and family.

In their strategies of resistance to the male power hierarchy the actions of the labour ward midwives echoed those of the industrial workers studied by Pollert (1981). In this study, she describes the actions of some of the older women in challenging the male authority as 'playing at turning the tables'. These strategies included addressing some of the younger male superiors in an overtly familial way, almost like sons or brothers. But as Pollert argues, this resistance is collusive as it never overtly challenges the basis for authority but reinforces the gendered family relationship. The resistance of the midwives also tended to centre upon fringe actions such as the taking-down of notices and the deliberate non-referral to the 'junior' male authority of the SHO.

So although women may experience the same working structures as men, they experience them differently. For instance, the underlying reasons and motivations for working the night shift in the labour ward came out of a set of specifically female obligations and social rules. Therefore, 'family' women 'chose' to work nights because it fitted in with domestic arrangements for child care and use of the car, and yet paradoxically, they felt that night work gave them more autonomy and power on the ward. In other words, for these women workers, the increase in professional autonomy in the public sphere is coexistent with a lack of personal autonomy in the private sphere. It also illustrates the differential in power between midwifery and the masculinised medical profession in that it is only at the time at which the most powerful are exercising a real choice to be absent that midwives can more closely approximate to the ideal of the independent practitioner with specialised skills.

It is here that the analogy between the working practice of hospital midwifery and industrial production breaks down. For despite certain similarities with factory line production, the midwife is not an unskilled or relatively low-paid worker. Midwifery as a female occupation has a high status within the feminised semi-professions and is a relatively well-paid job within the female labour force. Midwifery is recognised as that comparatively rare phenomenon – a skilled female occupation. Indeed with its almost exclusive female composition midwifery can claim to be among the 'aristocracy of female labour'. No other feminised occupation, not even nursing or teaching, can claim quite the legitimation of skill as its defining characteristic. This now leads us to an examination of the social meaning of 'skill'. How exactly is skilled work defined?

■ What is skill?

The notion of skill which once seemed an unambiguous concept, has been the centre of much recent feminist work. This locates the label of skill firmly within the social construction framework of explanation. As Phillips and Taylor (1986:55) clearly state:

> Far from being an objective economic fact, skill is often an ideological category imposed on certain types of work by virtue of the sex and power of the workers who perform it.

Cockburn (1990), in her study of the printing industry, shows how certain categories of work became defined as skilled and therefore the exclusive preserve of men. Rubery and Wilkinson (1979) showed that, within the manufacture of paper boxes and cartons, differentials of male and female work, pay and 'skill' were artificially created. Women making boxes on hand-fed machines were defined as unskilled labour, whereas men producing cartons on automated machines were classed as semi-skilled. The application of the label of skill had no relationship to the amount of dexterity, concentration or training involved.

This 'sexualisation' of skill labels as Phillips and Taylor term it, has made possible the segregation of male and female workers into separate spheres. The 'skilled' work, so defined, then becomes a predominantly male preserve and is hedged around by entry restrictions and barriers against intrusion by outsiders. Most women and men work in jobs which are predominantly either female or male (Hakim, 1978) and therefore whole collective occupational identities are constructed into gender hierarchies often legitimised by claims to skill. This occupational segregation which has been a feature of industrial and manufacturing production throughout this century (Gluckman, 1990; Walby, 1986) applies, of course, to the production site of birth – the labour ward.

This definition of skill as a gendered category and not an objective factual reality creates an alternative perspective on the differential skills possessed by the medical profession and midwives. In this situation the gendered skill hierarchies could be categorised as in Table 8.1.

In this description of the socially constructed categories of skill, the definition of normal and abnormal birth is, of course, crucial to the distinction between skilled and semi-skilled work. It marks the boundary upon which the whole professional hierarchy of skill is legitimised. Likewise the acquisition of an extension of knowledge by the unskilled workers will challenge the directly experienced and general everyday control exercised by the semi-skilled.

This perhaps explains the acknowledged antagonism articulated by some midwives towards the representation of 'skilled' and knowledgeable women in organisations like the NCT. They represent a challenge to these imposed categories of skill and authority structures.

So far we have viewed 'skill' as an ideological category which often disguises the reality of hierarchies based upon gender (and class). But is this just the *effect* which definitions of skill have produced or indeed were constructed for? Or is there a definable entity called 'a skill', however this is categorised and used to build hierarchies? Is there a skill of midwifery which perhaps has become marginalised historically by changes in the processes of production?

Table 8.1   Gendered skill hierarchies in a maternity unit

Skilled work – obstetricians and doctors

Area of practice	Abnormal birth – an unnatural and hazardous process
Main skills	Definition of hazard; technical expertise and application of scientific knowledge
Autonomy	Wide ranging encompassing all other workers in labour process
Place in hierarchy	Dominant
Other attributes	External professional objectivity

Semi-skilled work – midwifery

Area of practice	Normal birth – a natural process
Main skills	Ability to detect change to abnormal and limits to own skill
Autonomy	Limited – control over unskilled labour
Place in hierarchy	Middle
Other attributes	Experienced carer and supporter of women

Unskilled work – mother

Area of practice	Own labour
Main skills	None
Autonomy	Subordinate
Place in hierarchy	Lowest
Other attributes	Ability to obey orders

■ The deskilling debate

Martin (1991) has also taken up this metaphor of the birth process as mechanical production and argues that midwifery, like other occupations since industrialisation, has become increasingly deskilled. This deskilling process Braverman (1966) saw as an inevitable and essential part of the development of capitalist technological production. But groups of workers who have been affected by this process, have historically attempted to set up resistance to it. From the early Luddites who attempted to smash the machines which threatened their livelihood to the Wapping dispute of the early 1990s, a craft resistance to the process of deskilling with its accompanying loss of economic power and social status has been undertaken. Martin, writing from an American perspective, argues that a way of reasserting the skill of the midwife is for the site of birth to be changed. In other words, a return to a predominantly home birth system would restore the position and power of the midwife. This must be a familiar argument to anyone who has read articles in midwifery journals, feminist literature and indeed in some parts of the popular press. But is this a tenable position?

Unlike other male-based crafts which were highly prized and rewarded and which have become technologically deskilled, midwifery was a low-status and rather stigmatised occupation before professionalisation. Even after the Registration Act in 1902, midwifery had a long and difficult struggle to establish itself as a respectable and desirable occupation for women. It was given a degree of financial security and a position in public service in 1936, and after hospitalisation it became a good career move for the ambitious nurse, and consequently the rewards in terms of status improved.

So there is a basic contradiction in the deskilling argument. On the one hand, technological interventionist techniques and hospitalisation have undoubtedly altered the craft-skill base of midwifery, but at the same time, they have enabled midwifery to claim a recognisable occupational space within professional health care. Has then 'traditional' midwifery become as obsolete as hand-loom weaving or hot-metal print-setting? Or can it be revived within a different site of production?

It is often argued by midwives that it is possible to rediscover the 'real' skills which have become lost or hidden in recent medicalised childbirth. But even if this were so, the basic problem still remains, if skill is an *ideological* category within gendered power structures then is it not possible (or even probable) that the 'real skill' of midwifery will remain in a subordinated position within professional hierarchies, simply because it is possessed by women? As Phillips and Taylor state, 'skilled work is work that women don't do'. Or can midwifery overcome this ideological placing? Would the resiting of birth from the hospital setting merely provoke a *redefining* of skill within the existing set of power relations? This is a question to which we will return later in this chapter.

■ Deskilled or reskilled?

The argument about deskilling has another interesting dimension. I (SCH) trained as a midwife in the early 1970s and shortly after qualifying as a registered nurse undertook midwifery training. I worked in a very progressive consultant obstetric unit where modern technological intervention was highly prized. As a student I learnt the new skills of applying a fetal scalp electrode, I became adept at reading the recordings of the fetal heart monitor and I learnt to interpret the patterns of contractions derived from the use of the highly invasive intra-uterine catheter. As a 'high-technology' intensive-care 'nurse' I learnt how to flush out intra-uterine catheters blocked with amniotic fluid and vernix and sterilise the highly sensitive transducer. I was able to prepare a trolley for the doctor to perform fetal blood sampling. I could safely sterilise the equipment and ensure that the light source designed to illuminate the fetal scalp was in good working order. I learnt the new skill of being 'Guardian of the Cardiff Pump'. I knew when it was safe to override the automatic system and when to reduce the rate at which syntocinon was administered. Then, as I became more senior I was allowed into the operating theatre; as I gained confidence and experience I was allowed to stand close by the operating surgeon and watch the Sister pass him the instruments. When I qualified I felt that I had reached the pinnacle of technical proficiency when I too was allowed to scrub up and assist the surgeon by passing the correct instrument.

I learnt very little about women, very little about physiological birth and even less about developing my interpersonal and communication skills.

It was some years later after the high-technology birth of my own two children that I joined the ranks of the part-time midwives in a smaller maternity unit. At night, unsupported by medical staff but enriched by experienced midwives I began to learn the art of midwifery. I became re-skilled. My professional education had prepared me to be a doctor's assistant. I had been a maternity nurse in every sense of the word and knew very little about midwifery. With the support of some 'old hands' or expert practitioners, I discovered the skill of being a midwife and began to experience the power of professional practice. For the first time I began to understand the physiology of normal birth and believed in it.

I was not deskilled as a result of the high-technology 1970s but I acquired the nursing skills that were relevant to that era. Those skills had very little relevance for today's midwife or even for the midwife who was working alone or at night. I had become a skilled intensive-care delivery-room nurse, but I knew and understood very little of what women wanted. It was in the late 1980s that I became a midwife, 'with woman', and a confident competent practitioner of the art and science of midwifery.

Was it the move to hospital birth and the acquisition of the new skills of 'intensive-care delivery-room nurse' that deskilled today's midwife and was it also somewhere on that journey that midwives lost their ability to be 'with women' and communicate with women? When women had their babies at home they did not complain about lack of continuity of care or lack of choice or of lack of control. What they wanted was the assumed safety of the hospital and pain relief.

■ Where next for midwives and midwifery?

In 1992, the House of Commons Health Committee's Second Report into the Maternity Services (Chairman Nicholas Winterton) said that the key measure of the success of the maternity services in terms of their effectiveness and appropriateness would be in the responses from those who used them. In the chapter entitled 'What Women Want' it is reported that three main themes emerged from the evidence presented to the committee by women. These themes were the need for continuity of care, the desire for choice of care and place of delivery and the right to control over their own bodies at all stages of pregnancy and birth. Hence continuity, choice and control became the key words of the report. The ethnographic study presented in the preceding chapters has reflected similar themes.

■ Control?

The study of midwifery care at the Valley Maternity Hospital has revealed aspects of power and control. It has considered the way in which midwives have attempted to control their environment as well as women and the medical staff. The study has considered the midwives' view of real and unreal work and how through the 'Rules of Admission' they have attempted to slow down the production line. It is evident in this section of the study that the women who were recipients of the care at Valley Maternity Hospital had very little, if any, control over the process of birth.

Sheila Kitzinger in her evidence to the Health Committee said:

> Women who feel they can retain control over what is happening to them during birth, who understand the options available and are consulted about what they prefer, are much more likely to experience birth as satisfying than those who are merely at the receiving end of care, however kindly that care.

The women in this study appeared to have very low expectations for the experience of birth, indeed one was reported to evaluate her experience of birth by saying 'I am still here and I've got a son. How can I ask for anything more?'

Section 100 of the Health Committee Report concluded that:

> the experience of the hospital environment too often deters women from asserting control over their own bodies and too often left them feeling that, in retrospect, they did not have the best labour and delivery they could have hoped for.

This conclusion is supported in the ethnographic study but the implied solution must be challenged. There is very little evidence as yet to suggest that changing the site of birth will result in women being able to assert greater control over their own bodies. Women, because they are women, have the greatest difficulty in asserting themselves. When they are women in pain, in labour, lying horizontally and without even the protection of their undergarments, for them to attempt to control what is happening to them is very difficult if not impossible.

■ Continuity of carer?

The second major theme of the ethnographic study related to the issue of continuity of carer. It has explored the organisation of maternity care at the Valley Maternity Hospital and how that organisation impinged on the women's experience of birth. The research considered many aspects of continuity of care and carer and in particular the effects of the disruption in the care of women at the time of a shift handover.

As early as 1970 the Peel Report, which recommended the move towards 100% hospital birth stated:

> Continuity of care is a question raised several times in evidence and as such the concept is indisputably a good one.

However, it went on to say that with the complexity of modern organisations, it would be unrealistic for women to expect to have a continuous personal relationship with one midwife. It recommended that care be provided by teams of consultants, GPs and midwives. Later in 1980, the Social Services Committee Report (Chairman Mrs R. Short) stated in its section 'Humanising the Service':

> We recognise the difficulty of providing continuity of care throughout pregnancy and labour, but consider a measure of it can be attained by better organisation.

In 1992, the Health Committee Report stated:

> There is a strong desire amongst women for the provision of continuity of care and carer throughout pregnancy and childbirth, and that the majority of them regard midwives as the group best placed and equipped to provide this (para. 49).

and in paragraph 191:

> The evidence we have received suggests that the importance of continuity of care needs underlining very heavily for the professionals who are involved in delivering the maternity services of the NHS.

The fieldwork interviews for the ethnographic study explored the midwives' views and analysed their feelings about continuity of care. There is a clear conflict between the views expressed by the midwives in the study and the conclusion reached in Section 49 of the Health Committee Report.

Yet in 1992 continuity of care remained a major issue and the problem was no closer to being solved. The Institute of Manpower Studies Report, 'Mapping Team Midwifery' (Wraight *et al.*,1993) disappointedly explained that more than one quarter of the team midwifery schemes set up in 1990 had been discontinued by 1993.

Continuity of care is a recurring theme in much of the literature about birth. Yet in 1993 the Department of Health's Expert Maternity Group in its vision of 'A Comprehensive Maternity Service' (pp. 102–3) appears to weaken the previous resolve to provide continuity of care. It states:

> It is not clear from the evidence just how important, in itself, continuity of care is to most women.

and later:

> Continuity of care is most easily provided by one profession but in most cases, it is unlikely to be achieved and in practice there will be a spectrum of continuity. Within that lies the idea of continuity of care which implies that the woman should have the chance to build a relationship of trust with those looking after her throughout pregnancy, and that one of them should be available especially at crucial times such as the birth.

The Report argues that many of the current problems occur when communication breaks down between professionals and between them and the women and their families. It recommends as one solution amongst others that women be enabled to carry their own notes. It is highly unlikely that such a move would be sufficient to address the imbalance of power between midwives and women and between midwives and doctors nor to improve the adverse effects of discontinuity for the many hundreds of women who will find themselves outside a scheme which offers continuity of care. Finally the report does recommend that continuity will probably be best provided by small teams of midwives with their own case loads working between hospital and community and linked to primary health care teams.

■ Choice?

The third theme of the Health Committee report relates to the issue of choice. In paragraph 51 it states:

> The committee received evidence from women and the organisations that represent them that the choices available are more often illusory than real. Even the most articulate and assertive women may have difficulty achieving maximum choice in their contact with the maternity services.

The ethnographic study has indicated that most of the women receiving care at the Valley Maternity Hospital also had very little choice and indeed they often appeared as compliant passengers in the birth process. These passive women were the ones to whom something happened when they handed total responsibility for their well-being to the health-care workers around them. They had little knowledge in order to make choices and few opportunities existed to increase their knowledge. They were admitted to an alien environment, disrobed, identified, classified, washed, labelled, delivered and then 'washed and warded'. There was little evidence of choice, little continuity of carer, no control over their environment or their part in the labour process. The midwives were kind but were part of a system which for much of the time controlled their actions.

It would be easy to assume that these women were content with their care. There were apparently few complaints and clearly limited knowledge of what could have been. Realistic choice depends on having sufficient information on the alternatives that are actually available.

■ Communication?

This study has sadly demonstrated that the key issues of control, continuity and choice were in essence issues of communication. The women at Valley Maternity Hospital were without doubt rendered powerless by the system. The communication patterns were established in order to further the main goal of 'getting through the work'. Whilst the midwives were supportive, kind and technically proficient, the site of the birth process had reduced this crucial life event to a production-line system. Communication was a major issue that coloured the quality of the birth experience for most women.

Martin (1990) in her survey of the Maternity Services reports:

> At all stages of maternity care, the quality of communication between women and the professional staff was a crucial determinant of satisfaction with care.

When the professional staff are compelled to 'get through the work' and give care in a mechanical and task-orientated manner the opportunities for effective one-to-one communication with women are lost. There is no doubt that improving the continuity of the carer will improve the quality of communication. In the 'Know your Midwife' Report (Flint and Poulengeris, 1987) women in the scheme were more likely to be satisfied with their care and felt more in control of their labour than women who received traditional care.

Martin (1990) also found that continuity of care appeared to have significant implications for the woman's satisfaction with communication between her and the health professional.

There is now extensive evidence available in support of improving continuity of carer, e.g. The 'Know your Midwife' Report, The House of Commons Health Committee Report, *Mapping Team Midwifery*, *Changing Childbirth*. There is no doubt that one of the basic arguments for improving continuity of care is that it will inevitably result in improved communications between women and midwives.

Caroline Flint, writing in *Pregnancy Care in the 1990s*, says:

> Women have been asking to be looked after during labour by someone who has given them antenatal care and whom they have been able to get to know.

Even in 1993 communication is still a major issue in maternity care with Part II of *Changing Childbirth* being devoted to a Survey of Good Communication Practice in the Maternity Services, with the problem being far from solved.

■ New site: old problems?

The key issue to consider at this stage is whether moving the site of birth from hospital to home will address the main areas of concern in today's midwifery practice. It has been suggested that it is poor communication that leads women to be dissatisfied with the maternity services. It is this dissatisfaction that is expressed in feelings of frustration with the lack of continuity of carer, lack of choice through inadequate information and lack of control of the whole of the birth process. Will home birth or even *domino* (an abbreviation for domiciliary in and out scheme: where the woman is cared for mainly at home by a community midwife but comes to the hospital for the birth of the baby, and the woman then goes home a few hours later) and similar arrangements result in improvements in continuity, improved choice and greater control? What then would be the benefits to women of a change in the site of birth?

■ Women as winners?

There is no doubt that any scheme of care other than that described in this study would be likely to improve on continuity of carer. Most schemes described in the literature and especially in a planned home birth will result in the women meeting the midwife in advance of labour. Improved continuity of carer is more likely to improve communication between women and midwives. If the woman has established a relationship of trust with the midwife it is likely that she will be better informed and more able to make choices about all aspects of her care.

There is also no doubt that any birth that takes place away from a consultant obstetric unit will be less likely to involve unnecessary medical interventions. Prentice and Lind (1987), for example, in their review of all previous studies of fetal monitoring in labour, show that the only effect that electronic fetal monitoring has on birth statistics is to increase the rate of birth by Caesarian section.

It can also be argued that if the place of birth is the woman's home and as such her territory she is more likely to be in control of the birth process. As Farrar (1993) writing in the *AIMS Journal* explains:

Giving birth to a baby should be a wonderful time to look back on with delight and joy. If you want a calm, relaxed and in-control start to your baby's life give birth at home.

She goes on to offer a word of caution:

There is only one BUT, which is you must want it 200 per cent to achieve it.

Questions must also be asked about midwives. Can a generation of midwives trained in the world of obstetric intervention and medicalised birth and who have only ever worked in a hospital environment where they have had complete control over much of what happens, adapt and help turn women into winners? Will the midwives be willing and able to respond to the change in the focus of control or will they, like some other professionals, for example, Health Visitors, take control of the home environment and insist in making it like hospital?

According to Beech (1992):

> Giving birth at home in the company of your loved ones, in your own way and in your own time, can be an experience that enriches and strengthens the growing family.

As we have seen, the move to hospital birth was closely associated with availability of analgesia. Women giving birth at home in the 1990s, can also have free access to inhalation analgesia and other intramuscular analgesics as well as all other methods of pain relief. Those who have experienced home birth argue that they can cope better with the contractions and need less pain relief in the relaxed atmosphere of home, where they can eat and drink and are free to assume a variety of positions (Farrar, 1993).

Ultrasonic scanning and electronic fetal monitoring are also available at home and arrangements can be made to transmit fetal-heart recordings via the telephone lines if an expert second opinion is required.

Grant (1989) makes the following interesting point:

> Use of continuous electronic fetal monitoring changes the delivery room into an intensive care unit. The midwife takes on a more technical role with doctors becoming more centrally involved with routine care. The presence of a monitor may also change the relationship between the woman and her partner on one hand and the woman, midwife and doctor on the other.

and

> A fetal-heart monitor should be an adjunct to personal care not a substitute for it.

Home birth may result in women being winners in more ways than one. If the protagonists are to be believed, the benefits are many.

■ Women as losers?

Savage (1992) argues that home birth results in women feeling safe, relaxed and in control. She argues against herding women together in large understaffed places to which women must travel once labour has begun. She explains that expectant animals choose a quiet dark place for giving birth. However, her colleagues at the Royal College of Obstetricians and Gynaecologists do not share her views. Their press release issued on 6 August 1993 in response to the publication of *Changing Childbirth* states:

> Home confinement is suggested to be a reasonable option for some women. The College's view is that this is not a safe alternative to delivery in properly equipped surroundings. While we accept that some women will choose to have their babies at home, we do not think that the Report gives a realistic account of the consequences should a major change in policy occur.

The debate on safety continues with opinions firmly fixed on both sides. Why such intense discussion centres on an event which only affects the lives of some 1 per cent of the childbearing population is interesting in itself. Clearly women, midwives, GPs and obstetricians have much to gain and much to lose if the site of birth changes.

The loss, it seems, centres on the risk of home birth and the antagonists believe that the costs outweigh the benefits.

However, Campbell and MacFarlane (1987) as yet unchallenged, and after an extensive review of the maternity statistics concluded:

> There is no evidence to support the claim that the safest policy is for all women to give birth in hospital.

and

> Perhaps the most persistent and striking feature of the debate about where to be born, however, is the way in which policy has been formed with little reference to the evidence.

Has a woman anything else to lose if she chooses a home birth? First and foremost she will have been well-informed of the perceived risks of her decision. She may lose her calm serenity as she weighs up the risk of this 'reckless action'. She is also at risk of losing the status attached to the transition to motherhood. The public act of 'going to hospital' will be missing and perhaps she will not feel it necessary to buy new night-clothes and slippers for a birth at home. She will be deprived of the traumatic 'rush to hospital' and perhaps of the public concern of her relatives and friends who will have no hospital to telephone. Will anyone send flowers to her home? Perhaps there is a danger of losing her once- (or twice-) in-a-lifetime opportunity to be the centre of attraction. Perhaps she will be expected to resume her everyday duties that much sooner and will miss out on the extra attention of acting out the 'sick role'.

To some women the opportunity to acknowledge and respect the authority of the male doctor will be a missing ingredient in her home-birth experience. Deference to male authority figures remains a feature of many women's lives. Will birth (like skill) be redefined from an extraordinary event within the public sphere to an everyday occurrence in the private sphere and as one which is not mundane and normal but is 'what women do' – like housework? They receive neither acclaim or reward.

> Monument in York Minster to Mrs Hodgson, who died in 1636, at the age of 38, having borne 24 children:

> > The best of wives, who, having blest her husband with a numerous progeny of both sexes, at last in her 24th labour, she fell like a sentinel on duty, with the most perfect steadiness and tranquility of mind, in so early a period of life and such unfaded bloom of beauty, that she had the appearance rather of a virgin than of the mother of so many children.

> (Footnote: Astonishingly for that era, no fewer than 17 of her children survived to adulthood.)

Home birth may result in more losers than was first imagined. A change in the site of birth is only likely to benefit women by improving the continuity of care. It is reasonable to suppose that by getting to know a midwife, or at least a small team of midwives, a woman is likely to be better informed and be more able to make choices about her care. The question of control is less clear: there is little evidence to suggest that merely moving the site of birth will increase women's control over the birth process.

Finally some of the public drama of the occasion may be also lost in the process.

■ Midwives as winners or losers?

There are many midwives who are anxious to move away from the highly medicalised hospital-based style of care. Indeed the Association of Radical Midwives have amongst their objectives:

> to re-establish the confidence of the midwife in her own skills, to encourage midwives in their support of women's active participation in birth and to reaffirm the need for midwives to provide continuity of carers.

These midwives will obviously welcome the autonomy and freedom offered by home birth which will enable them to make full use of their skills and knowledge in enhancing the process of birth. They see the future as the opportunity for them to acquire status, respect and according to the Royal College of Midwives (1993) an enhanced pay structure.

But is this a simplification of a very complex set of conditions? As we have seen, 'skill' is not an unambiguous concept but a gendered category, and it is possible that the 'midwife's own skills' could in fact become redefined within the existing gendered professional structures.

It could therefore be argued that the present system of power relations will not be eradicated but merely rearranged into separate but unequal spheres and labour markets. In other words, could the future redefined categories appear as in Table 8.2?

Table 8.2   Reasons for arranging birth in hospital or at home

---

Hospital births – dominant sphere

Abnormal
Requires technical (male) skill and expertise
Midwife/maternity nurse subordinate to doctor
Skill categories remain

Home births – subordinate sphere

Normal and natural birth
Requires midwifery skills and experience
Midwife and woman in control

Hospital births will retain their connotations of 'skill' simply because the male-based professional hierarchies will practise there. Home will be the place where 'women do what women do'. This is the situation in other areas of social life, for instance, cooking and catering. Home cooking may be highly praised but the ordinary plain cook who regularly turns out three meals a day for a family does not occupy the high ground of the professional chef (usually male) who creates meals in the public site of a restaurant for high rewards and status.

Could midwifery, then, far from gaining in professional status because of increased autonomy actually lose out simply because that autonomy will become redefined within the existing set of ideological assumptions regarding both the primacy of the public over the private sphere and also the gender-based hierarchy of 'skill'?

There are other problems, too, regarding the organisation of a home-based workload for midwives. The Department of Health 'Expert Maternity Group' Report *Changing Childbirth* offers this sobering warning:

Making continuity of carer a reality will require a substantial degree of flexibility from midwives and their managers. Some midwives will welcome the opportunity to develop their skills more fully and will be able to adjust their personal lives so that they can be available when a woman needs them. For other midwives this will not be the case.

The Report goes on to argue that when midwives accept more responsibility their terms of employment, including remuneration received may need to be reviewed. It follows therefore, that if some midwives are prevented from participating in this move to greater continuity of carer (perhaps by small children or caring for elderly relatives) then they will earn less than those able to be fully involved. *Mapping Team Midwifery* investigated team midwifery and explained that this was a very different style of working. The midwives in such schemes were required to be more flexible, work more on-call hours and have increased responsibility. The authors comment that such factors can cause difficulties to midwives with dependents, those working part-time and the newly qualified. Midwifery thus is in danger of creating an underclass of low-paid female workers who cannot, because of their family commitments, give the type of care the latest Government reports are recommending or, worse, creating a career open only to the single woman who is presumed to have no other life.

■ The future?

In conclusion, the reader may be left with the view that the events recorded and discussed in this ethnography are a sad reflection on current midwifery practice. I believe that it is only when midwives openly accept that the care described here is not satisfactory and acknowledge that in most instances it is they and not women who control birth, that we can begin to construct a clearer vision of the future.

Only when midwives start to see women as equal partners in the experience of birth and move towards being truly 'with women' will there be any real chance for care to be all that it could and should be.

Glossary of terms

Anti-D   A substance given by intramuscular injection to a woman whose blood group is rhesus negative. It is given after the birth of the baby to prevent or reduce the risk of rhesus incompatibility in subsequent pregnancies.

Apgar score   A method of scoring and assessing the baby's condition at birth. The higher the score, the better the baby's condition.

Breech presentation   A delivery where the baby's buttocks lie lowest in the pelvis.

Brow presentation   A head presentation where the head is deflexed so that the highest point on the forehead lies lowest in the pelvis. It is a possible cause of obstructed labour.

Cervix   The neck of the uterus.

Crowning   The moment during birth when the widest diameters of the fetal head have been born.

ECTG   Electro-cardiotogograph trace. A recording of the fetal heart rate and uterine activity.

EDD   Estimated date of delivery of the baby.

FMs   Fetal movements. These are counted by the woman and are used as a guide to fetal well-being.

Footling   In a breech presentation where the fetal foot lies lowest in the pelvis.

FSE   Fetal scalp electrode – a device used to record the fetal heart rate. It is attached to the fetal head during a vaginal examination.

Fully   An abbreviation commonly used to describe the second stage of labour when the cervix was fully dilated.

Gravida   A pregnant woman.

Induction   A term used to mean the process whereby labour is artificially started using drugs.

IUGR   Intra-uterine growth retardation – a condition where the fetus *in utero* is not growing at the normal rate.

Multigravida   A pregnant woman who has previously had one or more pregnancies.

Multipara   A woman who has borne more than one child (often abbreviated to 'Multip.')

$N_2O + O_2$ Nitrous oxide and oxygen. An analgesic drug, a gas self-administered by the patient during labour.

NCT   National Childbirth Trust

NND   Neonatal Death – an infant that dies within the first week of life.

O-Neg   Refers to the woman's blood group.

Obs   Observations – an abbreviation for activities that include taking and recording the woman's blood pressure, pulse rate, respiratory rate, etc.

155

Para	Parous – having borne an infant.
PE	Pre-eclampsia, a disease of pregnancy.
Pethidine	A powerful analgesic drug given by intra-muscular injection to women in labour.
Prem	Pre-term – a baby born early, before thirty-six weeks gestation.
Primigravida	A woman pregnant for the first time.
Primiparous	Often abbreviated to 'primip' or 'prim'. Correctly means having borne one child. Often used to mean primigravida.
SB	Still birth.
Shoulder dystocia	Difficulty in delivering the baby's shoulders.
Show	A lay term for the plug of mucous lost from the cervix at the start of labour.
Speculum	An instrument used to examine the cervix and vagina.
SROM	Spontaneous Rupture of Membranes – when the bag of water around the baby breaks and water (amniotic fluid) is lost.
Stages of labour	
1st Stage	The onset of regular painful contractions and dilatation of the cervix.
2nd Stage	From full dilatation of cervix until delivery of the baby.
3rd Stage	From the birth of the baby until delivery of the placenta or afterbirth.
Syntocinon	A drug used to induce labour, given intravenously.
Syntometrine	A drug used to minimise the blood loss during the third stage of labour.
Vitamin K	A vitamin drug preparation given to babies at Valley Maternity Hospital to minimise the risks associated with haemorrhagic disease of the newborn.
VE	Vaginal Examination. Carried out by midwives and doctors for a variety of reasons, e.g. to confirm the onset of labour, to assess progress in labour, to rupture membranes, etc.

References

Balaskas, J. (1983) *Active Birth* (London: Unwin Paperbacks).

Bashford, A. (1993) 'The Sanitarian Discourse', paper given to the Women's Studies: Nursing History and Politics of Welfare Conference, Nottingham University, July 1993.

Becker, H. S., Everett, B., Hughes, G. and Strauss, A. L. (1961) *Boys in White: Student Culture in Medical School* (Chicago University Press).

Beech, B. A. L. (1992) 'Arranging a Birth at Home', *Association for Improvement in the Maternity Services (AIMS) Journal*, 4, 4, Winter 1992/93, p. 11.

Benner, P. (1984) *From Novice to Expert: Excellence and Power in Clinical Nursing Practice* (Menlo Park: Addison Wesley).

Berne, E. (1968) *Games People Play: The Psychology of Human Relationships* (Harmondsworth: Penguin).

Beynon, H. (1973) *Working for Ford* (Harmondsworth: Penguin).

Birth: 9000 Mothers Speak Out. Birth Survey 1986 Results, *Parents Magazine*, 128.

Blumer, J. (1954) 'What is Wrong with Social Theory?', *American Sociological Review*, 19, pp. 3–10.

Borhek, J. T. and Curtis, R. F. (1975) *A Sociology of Belief* (New York: Wiley).

Boyd, C. and Sellars, L. (1982) *The British Way of Birth* (London: Pan).

Braverman, H. (1966) *Labor and Monopoly Capital: The Degradation of Work in the 20th century* (New York: Monthly Review Place).

Campbell, J. (1923) *Training of Midwives – Report on Public Health and Medical Subjects*, no 21 (London: HMSO).

Campbell, R. and MacFarlane, A. (1987) *Where to be Born? The Debate and the Evidence* (Oxford: National Perinatal Epidemiology Unit) pp. 58–9.

Cartwright, A. (1967) *Patients and their Doctors – A Study of General Practice* (London: Routledge & Kegan Paul).

Cavendish, R. (1982) *Women on the Line* (London: Routledge & Kegan Paul).

Chamberlain, M. (1981) *Old Wives Tales; Their History, Remedies and Spells* (London: Virago).

Clarke, M. (1978) 'Getting Through the Work', in Dingwall, R. and McIntosh, J., *Readings in the Sociology of Nursing* (London: Churchill Livingstone).

Cockburn, C. (1990) *Brothers; Male Dominance and Technological Change* (London: Pluto Press).

Cowell, B. and Wainwright, D. (1981) *Behind the Blue Door; The History of the RCM 1851–1981* (London: Balliere Tindall).

Cronk, M. (1992) 'How Did We Get into this Mess in the First Place?', *Midwives Information and Resource Service Midwifery Digest* (March 1992) 2, 1, pp.6–8.

Craig, C., Rubery, J., Talling, R. and Wilkinson, F. (1980) *Abolition and After. The Paper Box Wages Council*, Research Paper by Labour Studies Group (London: Department of Employment).

Curtis, P.(1992) 'Supervision in Clinical Midwifery Practice', in Butterworth, T. and Faugier, J. (eds) (1992) *Clinical Supervision & Mentorship in Nursing* (London: Chapman & Hall).

Davidoff, L. and Hall, C. (1987) *Family Fortunes: Men and Women of the English Middle Class 1700–1850* (London: Hutchinson).

Davies, C. (1988) 'The Health Visitor as Mother's Friend; A Woman's Place in Public Health 1890–1914', *Social History of Medicine*, 1, 1, pp. 39–59.

Davies, M.L. (ed.) (1978) *Maternity Letters from Working Women, Women's Cooperative Guild* (London: Virago).

Davin, A. (1978) 'Imperialism and Motherhood', *History Workshop 5*, pp. 9–65.

Department of Health, *Changing Childbirth, August 1993*: Part I, Report of the Expert Maternity Group. Part II, Survey of Good Communication Practice in Maternity Services (London: HMSO).

Dex, S. (1985) *The Sexual Division of Work* (Brighton: Harvester Wheatsheaf).

Dingwall, R., Rafferty, A. and Webster, C. (1991) *An Introduction to the Social History of Nursing* (London: Routledge).

Dingwall, R. W. J. (1977) 'Atrocity Stories and Professional Relationships', *Sociology of Work and Occupations*, 4, pp. 371–96.

Dingwall, R. (1992) '"Don't mind him – he's from Barcelona": Qualitative methods in health studies', in Daly, J., McDonald, I. and Willis, E. (eds) *Researching Health Care, Designs, Dilemmas, Disciplines* (London and New York: Tavistock/Routledge).

Donnison, J. (1977) *Midwives and Medical Men* (London: Heinemann).

Douglas, M. (1976) *Purity and Danger: An Analysis of Concepts of Pollution and Taboo* (London: Routledge & Kegan Paul).

Drayton, S. and Rees, C. (1984) 'They Know What They're Doing', *Nursing Mirror (Midwifery Forum)* 159, 3, pp. iv–viii.

Ehrenreich, B. and English, D. (1973) *For Her Own Good; 150 years of Expert Advice to Women* (Writers' and Readers' Publishing Cooperative, London).

Emerson, J. P. (1970) 'Behaviour in Private Places: Sustaining Definitions of Reality in Gynaecological Examinations', in Dreitsel, H. P. (ed.) *Patterns of Communicative Behaviour* (London: Collier Macmillan).

Etzioni, A. (1969) *The Semi-Professionals and their Organizations* (New York: Free Press).

Everhart, R. B. (1977) 'Between Stranger and Friend: Some Consequences of 'Long Term' Fieldwork in Schools', *American Educational Research Journal* 14, 1, pp. 1–15.

Farrar, J. (1993) 'Home Alone? Yes – It is Possible', *Association for the Improvement of Maternity Services (AIMS) Quarterly Journal*, 5, 2, Summer 1993, p. 11.

Field, P.A. (1980) 'Four Nurses: Perspectives on Nursing in a Community Health Setting', unpublished Ph.D. Thesis, University of Alberta, Edmonton.

Field, P.A. and Morse, J.M. (1985) *Nursing Research: The Application of Qualitative Approaches* (London: Croom Helm).

Finch, J. (1984) 'The Deceit of Self-help; Pre-School Playgroups and Working-class Mothers', *Journal of Sociological Policy*, 13, 1, pp. 1–20.

Firth, R. (1981) 'Routines in a Tropical Disease Hospital', in Davis, A. and Horobin, G. (eds) *Medical Encounters* (London: Croom Helm).

Flint, C. (1986) 'The "Know Your Midwife" Scheme', *Nursing Times*, 14 May 1986, p. 26.

Flint, C. (1992) 'The Basis of a Midwifery Team: Continuity of Care', Chapter 13 in Chamberlain, G. and Sander, L. (eds) *Pregnancy Care in the 1990s* (Lancashire, UK, and New Jersey, USA: Parthenon Publishing Group).

Flint, C. and Poulengeris, P. (1987) 'The "Know Your Midwife" Report', 49 Peckarmans Wood, Sydenham Hill, London.

Foucault, M. (1977) *Discipline and Punish: The Birth of the Prison* (Harmondsworth: Penguin).

Fox, N. (1992) *The Social Meaning of Surgery* (Milton Keynes: Open University Press).

Franklin, B. (1974) *Patient Anxiety of Admission to Hospital* (London: Royal College of Nursing).

Freilich, M. (1970) 'Mohawk Heroes and Trinidadian Peasants', in Freilich, M. (ed.) *Marginal Natives: Anthropologists at Work* (New York: Harper & Row).

Friedson, E. (1970) *Profession of Medicine; A Study of the Sociology of Applied Knowledge* (New York: Harper & Row).

Friedson, E. (1977) 'The future of professionalism', in Stacey, M. and Reid, M. (eds) *Health and the Division of Labour* (London: Croom Helm).

Garcia, J. and Garforth, S. (1989) 'Labour & Delivery Routines in English Consultant Units' *Midwifery*, 5, 4, Dec 1989, pp. 155–62.

Garforth, S. and Garcia, J. (1987) 'Admitting – a Weakness or a Strength', *Midwifery*, 3, 1, March 1987, pp. 10, 23.

Garmonikow, E. (1984) 'Sexual Division of Labour – The Case of Nursing', in Kuhn, A. and Wolpe, A., *Feminism and Materialism* (London: Routledge & Kegan Paul).

Gerth, H. and Mills, C. W. (1970) *From Max Weber* (London: Routledge & Kegan Paul).

Glaser, B. and Strauss, A. (1967) *The Discovery of Grounded Theory* (Chicago, Illinois: Aldine).

Gluckman, M. (1990) *Women Assemble* (London: Routledge).

Granshaw, L. and Porter, R. (eds) (1990) *The Hospital in History* (London: Routledge).

Grant, A. (1989) 'Monitoring the fetus during labour' (Ch.54. p. 878) in *Effective Care in Pregnancy and Childbirth*, vol. 2 Childbirth, edited by Iain Chalmers, Murray Enkin and Marc J. N. C. Keirse (Oxford, New York and Toronto: Oxford University Press).

Gumperz, J. (1981) 'Conversational Inference and Classroom Learning', in Green, J. L. and Wallat, C. (eds) *Ethnography and Language in Educational Settings* (Norwood, NJ: Ablex).

Hakim, C. (1978) 'Sexual divisions in the labour force', *Employment Gazette*, November.

Hall, C. (1985) 'Private persons versus public someones; class gender and politics in England 1780–1850', in C. Steedman *et al.*, *Language, Gender and Childhood* (London: Routledge & Kegan Paul).

Hammersley, M. (1983b) 'Introduction: Reflexivity and Naturalism', in Hammersley (ed.) *The Ethnography of Schooling: Methodological Issues* (Driffield: Nafferton).

Hammersley, M. and Atkinson, P. (1983) *Ethnography: Principles in Practice* (London: Tavistock).

Health Committee Report, Session 1991–92 (Chairman: Mr Nicholas Winterton) *Maternity Services* vol. 1 (London: HMSO, 1992).

Hearn, J. (1982) 'Notes on Patriarchy, Professionalism and the Semi-professions', *Sociology*, vol. 16.

Hearn, J. (1987) *The Gender of Oppression* (Brighton: Harvester Wheatsheaf).

Honigsbaum, C. (1979) *The Division in British Medicine; A History of the Separation of General Practice and Hospital Care, 1911–1968* (London: Kogan Page).

Hughes, D. (1988) 'When Nurse Knows Best: Some Examples of Nurse–Doctor Interaction in a Casualty Department', *Sociology of Health and Illness*, 10, 1, pp. 1–22.

Hughes, E. C. (1971) *The Sociological Eye: Selected Papers* (Chicago and New York: Aldine Athaton).

Humphries, S. and Gordon, P. (1993) *A Labour of Love* (London: Sidgwick & Jackson).

Jeffrey, R. (1979) 'Normal Rubbish: Deviant Patients in Casualty Departments', *Sociology of Health and Illness* 1, pp. 98–107.

Johnson, T. (1972) *Professions and Power* (London: Macmillan).

Kelly, M.P. and May, D. (1982) 'Good and Bad Patients: A Review of the Literature and a Theoretical Critique', *Journal of Advanced Nursing*, 7, pp. 147–56.

Kenny, C. (1993) 'Power and Knowledge: The case of the EN', unpublished paper presented at Nursing, Women's History and the Politics of Welfare Conference, Nottingham University, July 1993.

Kirkham, M. (1983) 'Admission in Labour: Teaching the Patient to be Patient', *Midwives Chronicle*, February 1983.

Kirkham, M. (1983) 'Labouring in the Dark: Limitations on Giving of Information to enable Patients to Orientate themselves to the Likely Events and Timescale of Labour', in Wilson-Barnet, J. (ed.) *Nursing Research: Ten Studies in Patient Care* (Chichester: Wiley) pp. 81–9.

Kirkham, M. (1989) 'Midwives and Information-giving during labour', in Robinson, S. and Thomson, A.N. (eds) *Midwives Research and Childbirth*, vol. 1 (London: Chapman & Hall).

Kirkham, M. (1992) 'Labouring in the Dark', in Abbott, P. and Sapsford, R. *Research into Practice: A Reader for Nurses and the Caring Professions* (Milton Keynes: Open University Press).

Kitzinger, S. (1978) 'Pain in Childbirth', *Journal of Medical Ethics*, 4, January, pp. 119–21.

Kreckel, R. (1980) 'Unequal Opportunities Structure and the Labour Market Segmentation', *Sociology*, 4, pp. 525–50

Leap, N. and Hunter, B. (1993) *The Midwife's Tale* (London: Scarlett Press).

Leininger, M. (1969) 'Ethnoscience: A Promising Research Approach to Improve Nursing Practice', *Image: The Journal of Nursing Scholarship*, 3, 1, pp. 2–8.

Lewis, J. (1980) *Politics of Motherhood; Child and Maternal Welfare in England 1900–1939* (London: Croom Helm).

Lofland, J. (1971) *Analyzing Social Settings: A Guide to Qualitative Analysis* (Belmont, California: Wadsworth).

Lofland, J. and Lofland, L.H. (1984) *Analysing Social Settings: A Guide to Qualitative Observation and Analysis* (Belmont, California: Wadsworth) 2nd edn.

Loudon, I. (1986) 'Deaths in Childbed from 18th century to 1935', *Bulletin of History of Medicine*, 30, pp. 1–41.

Lutz, F.W. (1981) 'Ethnography – The Holistic Approach to Understanding Schooling', in Green, J.L. and Wallat, C. (eds) *Ethnography and Language in Educational Settings* (Norwood, New Jersey: Ablex).

Macfarlane, A. and Mugford, M. (1984) *Birth Counts – Statistics of Pregnancy and Childbirth* (London: HMSO).

Malinowski, B. (1922) *Argonauts of the Western Pacific* (London: Routledge & Kegan Paul). Quoted in Hammersley and Atkinson (1983).

Martin, C. (1990) 'How Do You Count Maternal Satisfaction? – A User-commissioned Survey of Maternity Services', in Helen Roberts (ed.) *Women's Health Counts* (London: Routledge).

Martin, E. (1991) *The Woman in the Body* (Milton Keynes: Open University Press).

Mass Observation (1945) *Britain and her Birth Rate* (London: John Murray).

Menzies, M. (1942) 'Hospital or Domiciliary Confinement?', *Lancet*, 11 July, pp. 35–8.

Ministry of Health (1924) *Maternal Mortality DHMS*, no. 26 (London: HMSO).

Ministry of Health (1937) *Report on Maternal Mortality*, CMD 5422 (London: HMSO).

Ministry of Health (1949) *Report of Working Party on Midwives* (London: HMSO).

Murcott, A. (1981) 'On the Typification of "Bad Patients" ', in Atkinson, P. and Heath, C. (eds) *Medical Work: Realities and Routines* (Guildford: Gower).

Nettleton, S. (1992) *Power, Pain and Dentistry* (Buckingham: OUP).

Nurses, Midwives and Health Visitors Act (1979) (Ch. 36) (London: HMSO).

Nursing Notes and Midwives Chronicle (1934) 'Operative Midwifery and the Use of Drugs', July, pp.109–10.

Oakley, A. (1980) *Women Confined* (Oxford: Martin Robertson).

Oakley, A. (1984) *The Captured Womb* (Oxford: Blackwell).

Oakley, A. (1989) 'Who Cares for Women? Science versus Love in Midwifery Today', *Midwives Chronicle*, July, pp. 214–21.

Office of Population, Census and Survey, *Birth Statistics: Review of the Registrar General on Birth and Patterns of Family Building in England and Wales* (1991) (London: HMSO).

Parsons, T. (1951) *The Social System* (Glencoe, Illinois: Free Press).

Parsons, T. (1954) *The Professions and Social Structure: Essays in Social Theory* (New York: Free Press).

Percival, R. (1970) 'Management of Normal Labour', *The Practitioner*, 1221, March, p. 204.

Phillips, A. and Taylor, B. (1986) 'Sex and Skill Waged Work', *Feminist Review* (London: Virago).

Pollert, A. (1981) *Girls, Wives and Factory Lives* (Basingstoke: Macmillan).

Porter, S. (1991) 'A Participant Observation Study of Power Relations between Nurses and Doctors in a General Hospital', *Journal of Advanced Nursing*, 16, pp. 728–35.

Porter, S. (1993) 'Critical Realistic Ethnography: The Case of Racism and Professionalism in a Medical Setting', *Sociology* 27, 4, pp. 591–609.

Powdermaker, H. (1966) *Stranger and Friend: The Way of an Anthropologist* (New York: Norton).

Prentice, A. and Lind, T. (1987) 'Fetal Heart Rate Monitoring During Labour – Too Frequent Intervention, Too Little Benefit', *Lancet*, 2, pp. 1375–77.

Raphael, W. (1969) *Patients and Their Hospitals* (London: King Edward's Hospital Fund for London).

RCOG (1944) *Report on a National Maternity Service* (London: Royal College of Obstetricians and Gynaecologists).

Reid, P. (1983) 'Review Article – A Feminist Sociological Imagination? Reading Anne Oakley', *Sociology, Health and Illness*, 5, pp. 83–93.

Richman, J. and Goldthorpe, W.O. (1977) 'When was your Last Period?', in Dingwall, R. *et al.*, *Health Care and Health Knowledge* (London: Croom Helm) p. 164.

Robinson, S., Golden, J. and Bradley, S. (1983) *A Study of the Role and Responsibilities of the Midwife*, Nursing Education Research Unit Report no. 1, 1984.

Rogers, C.R. (1983) *Freedom to learn for the 80s* (Columbus, Ohio: Charles E. Merrill).

Roth, J. (1963) *Timetables: Structuring the Passage of Time in Hospital Treatment and Other Careers* (New York: Bobbs Merill).

Roth, J. (1972) 'Some Contingencies of the Moral Evaluation and Control of the Clientele: The Case of the Hospital Emergency Service', *American Journal of Sociology*, 77, 5, March 1972.

Roth, J. (1978) 'Ritual and Magic in the Control of Contagion', in Dingwall, R. and McIntosh, J. (eds) *Readings in the Sociology of Nursing* (Ch. 10) (Edinburgh and London: Churchill Livingstone).

Royal College of Midwives (September 1993) 'Evidence to the Review Body for Nursing Staff, Midwives, Health Visitors and Professionals Allied to Medicine for 1994' (London: Royal College of Midwives).

Royal College of Obstetricians and Gynaecologists Press Release 6 August 1993, 'Changing Childbirth: Report of the Expert Group on Maternity Services', RCOG, 27 Sussex Place, Regents Park, London.

Rubery, J. and Wilkinson, F. (1979) 'Notes on the Nature of the Labour Process in the Secondary Sector', *Low Pay and Labour Market Segregation Conference Papers*, Cambridge.

Sandwell, J. (1993) Paper given at Conference, University of Nottingham.

Savage, W. (1992) 'Our free society ought to deliver choice on births', *Association for the Improvement of Maternity Services (AIMS) Quarterly Journal*, 4, 4, Winter 1992–3, pp. 15–16.

Savage, W. (1986) *A Savage Enquiry: Who Controls Childbirth?* (London: Virago).

Simpson, R. and Simpson, I. (1969) 'Women and Bureaucracy in the Semi-professions' in Etzoni, A. (ed.) (1969) *Semi Professions and Organisations* (New York: Free Press).

Smith, P. (1992) *Emotional Labour of Nursing* (Basingstoke: Macmillan).

Social Services Committee (Chairman: Mrs Renee Short) *2nd Report – Perinatal & Neonatal Mortality* (London: HMSO, 1980).

Spradley, J.P. (1979) *The Ethnographic Interview* (New York: Holt, Rinehart & Winston).

Spradley, J.P. (1980) *Participant Observation* (New York: Holt, Rinehart & Winston).

Spradley, J.P. and McCurdy, D. (1972) *The Cultural Experience: Ethnography in Complex Society* (Chicago: Science Research Associated).

Spring-Rice, M. (1939) *Working-Class Wives* (London: Virago).

Standing Maternity and Midwifery Advisory Committee (Chairman: Sir John Peel) *Domiciliary Midwifery and Maternity Beds Needs* (London: HMSO, 1970).

Stimpson, G. and Webb, B. (1975) *Going to See the Doctor: The Consultation Process in General Practice* (London: Routledge & Kegan Paul).

Strong, P. and Davis, A. (1978) 'Who's Who in Paediatric Encounters: Morality, Expertise and the Generation of Identity and Action in Medical Settings', in Davis, A. (ed.) *Relationships between Doctors and Patients* (Westmead: Takfield) pp. 51–2.

Sudnow, D. (1967) *Passing On: The Social Organisation of Dying* (Englewood Cliffs, New Jersey: Prentice Hall).

Symonds, A. (1991) 'Angels and Interfering Busybodies: The Social Construction of Two Occupations', *Sociology, Health and Illness*, 13, 2, pp. 249–69.

Tew, M. (1977) 'Where to be born?', *New Society*, 20 January, pp. 120–1.

Towler, J. and Bramall, J. (1986) *Midwives in History and Society* (Beckenham: Croom Helm).

United Kingdom Central Council for Nursing, Midwifery and Health Visiting (June 1992) *The Code of Professional Conduct* (London: UKCC).

United Kingdom Central Council for Nursing, Midwifery and Health Visiting (May 1986) *A Midwives Code of Practice for Midwives Practising in the United Kingdom* (London: UKCC).

United Kingdom Central Council For Nursing, Midwifery and Health Visiting (November 1991) *Statistical Analysis of the Council's Professional Register 1 April 1990 to 31 March 1991* (London: UKCC).

Walby, S. (1986) *Patriarchy at Work* (London: Polity Press).

Walker, J. (1972) 'The Changing Role of the Midwife', *International Journal of Nursing Studies 9*, pp. 85–94.

Walker, J. (1976) 'Midwife or Obstetric Nurse? Some Perceptions of Midwives and Obstetricians on the Role of the Midwife', *Journal of Advanced Nursing*, 1, pp. 129–39.

Walker, R. (1981) 'On the Uses of Fiction in Educational Research', in Smetherham, D. (ed.) *Practising Evaluation*. (Driffield: Nafferton).

Walkowitz, J. (1993) *City of Dreadful Delight; Narratives of Sexual Danger in late-Victorian London* (London: Virago).

Wilensky, H. (1964) 'The Professionalisation of Everyone', *American Journal of Sociology*, 70, pp. 137–48.

Willis, P. (1979) *Shopfloor Culture, Masculinity and the Wage Form, Working-Class Culture: Studies in History Theory* (London: Hutchinson).

Willmott, P. and Young, M. (1960) *Family and Kinship in East London* (Harmondsworth: Penguin).

Witz, A. (1992) *Professionals and Patriarchy* (London: Routledge & Kegan Paul).

Wraight, A., Ball, J., Seccombe, I. and Stock, J. (March 1991) *Mapping Team Midwifery – A Report to the Department of Health* (Brighton: Institute of Manpower Studies – Report No. 242).

Zerubavel, E. (1979) *Patterns of Time in Hospital Life* (Chicago and London: University of Chicago Press).

Index